# DEMYSTIFYING
# ACUPUNCTURE

## MODERN ANSWERS ABOUT ANCIENT MEDICINE

by Sina Leslie Smith, MS, MA, LAc, MD
Dipl. Ac. NCCAOM, FAAMA

Edited by Lil Barcaski

Published by: GWN Publishing
www.GWNPublishing.com

Cover Design: Larry Bak.

ISBN: 978-1-959608-77-6

*I dedicate this book to my mother,*
*Charlotte,*

*Who has never stopped believing in me*

*No matter what I decide to do next.*

# TABLE OF CONTENTS

# FOREWORD

## Q. Why write this book?

As a medical doctor and licensed acupuncturist with a clear enthusiasm for explaining how the body works, I get lots and lots of questions about acupuncture. Questions like "How does it work?" "What does it do?" and "What should I expect when I come in for treatment?" are common topics of conversation for me in the elevator, on an airplane, or in a coffee shop.

I have had the chance to practice answering these questions in many contexts: on my various websites, in newsletters, in lectures to the conventional medical community, and in the training of colleagues and student doctors. Like many acupuncturists, I have also had the privilege of helping people heal using this medicine and as such, have answered the questions of thousands of patients. Because so many people have the same questions, I decided to compile them together in this book.

## Q. Who am I to write this book?

I would like to acknowledge that I am an American white woman who is going to talk to you about acupuncture. My mother is Dutch and immigrated when she was 12 years old to the US. My father is an American of Scottish, German and Blackfeet Nation (Pikuni) descent. To my knowledge, I am not Chinese, Japanese, Korean or otherwise of Asian heritage or background. I have learned the traditional East Asian medical system in academic settings, while studying with various practitioners, in continuing education coursework, and at conferences. I have practiced it on my patients, on family and friends, on a few people sitting next to me on the plane in extreme pain or GI upset, and on myself since 2009.

While I moved to Los Angeles from Illinois specifically to learn this medicine from people of East Asian heritage, I recognize that this is not at all the same as having a lived familiarity of traditional East Asian medicine as a part of my culture. It is my hope that this book is not received as a way of taking an opportunity away from the persons who might speak from a place of cultural authority, nuance, or deeper wisdom because it is a part of their heritage. It is my sincere desire that my voice is supportive of that wisdom and not a detractor or replacement for it. Please see the list of books in the References section by authors who do speak from a space of cultural authority should you wish to learn from someone with a different voice and background than me.

I am grateful to my Asian and non-Asian teachers who have generously and patiently shared their knowledge, answered my questions, and guided me to the insights that I am about to share with you. I take full responsibility for any errors in my understanding, and welcome feedback on this book so that I can correct any misrepresentations or mistakes in future editions.

To that end, if you would like to point out any misunderstandings or errors in this book, please send me an email at DemystifyingAcupCorrections@SinaSmithMD.com. I welcome your feedback and wisdom and look forward to learning from you.

## Q. How to use this book.

This book is meant to be a quick reference guide for the general public and to increase general awareness and understanding of acupuncture and related therapies. It is intended to be accurate but also pithy. Therefore, it is by necessity relatively superficial in the face of an ancient medical system that encompasses thousands of years of thought and clinical practice. I have included only a few references specific to the book so as to avoid overwhelming the reader, while still providing places to go next should the reader be curious about a particular topic or about acupuncture in general. The References section has both references for the book and for more reading should you wish to do so.

In order to make it understandable to the general public, I have had to choose to use some generalizations that I would not necessarily use in other audiences. This is equivalent to saying "heel" to a non-medical person versus "calcaneus interdigitating with the cuboid bone and talus" to a medical professional. It is not intended to be a comprehensive textbook for conventional, integrative, or alternative practitioners looking to understand detailed mechanisms of action, scientific theory of acupuncture, or the history and evolution of traditional East Asian medical theory. Please see the References section for a list of journal articles and websites specifically for medical professionals.

Finally, please do not mistakenly use this book as a substitute for personal advice from a practitioner familiar with your concerns and your health history. Should you wish to find such a practitioner of traditional East Asian medicine in your community, I recommend looking for someone who is a licensed acupuncturist through your state's department of professional regulation or on the NCCAOM website. There is a long list of acupuncture-related organizations in the References section with the URLs for all of them. You can also, of course, ask around: one of your friends or colleagues is likely already seeing an acupuncturist that they can recommend to you.

## Q. What's with the capitalization?

When authors are speaking of a western concept of, for example, a liver, it is written with lowercase letters. It ("liver") means the physical structure of the squishy organ that lives on the right side of your abdomen under your ribcage. As an adjective (e.g. "liver function tests"), "liver" also refers to the functions of the liver organ: detoxification, making clotting factors, iron recycling and removal, etc.

When I am speaking of the traditional East Asian medicine concept of "Liver," it is written with a capital letter. "Liver" refers to the physical structure and functions of that same squishy liver organ, but also to the larger system of Zang and Fu organs, the Wood system, the channels, the acupoints, the spirit, etc. to which it belongs. It is bigger, if you will, than just the organ itself, so it gets a capital letter. Likewise, words like "Yin," "Yang," and "Qi" are commonly written with a capital letter. I have maintained that convention in this book.

# CHAPTER ONE

# WHAT ARE THE FOUNDATIONAL CONCEPTS OF ACUPUNCTURE?

## Q. What is Traditional East Asian Medicine (TEAM)?

Acupuncture is part of a whole-body system of medicine that originated in China at least 2,500 years ago. In recent history, this system has been called "Traditional Chinese Medicine" (TCM), but that term does not give credit to the other cultures (Japanese, Korean, Vietnamese, etc.) that developed, adopted, contributed to, and influenced acupuncture theory and practice in various ways. The term "Traditional East Asian Medicine" (TEAM) has been more recently applied to this medical system and is more inclusive of these other cultural influences on the medical system. But I fully acknowledge that it is also an imperfect descriptor. It also downplays the unique cultural differences in concept and style of the various traditional medicines. However, for the purposes of this book, I will use TEAM until a more acceptable term is conceived by and accepted by stakeholders in the acupuncture community and the cultural stakeholders from which acupuncture and the various forms of TEAM were conceived and developed.

The first textbook of TCM, the *Huang Di Nei Jing* ("Yellow Emperor's Inner Classic" or "Yellow Emperor's Cannon of Internal Medicine") is believed to have been compiled by many different scholars over approximately 500 years (100 BC to 400 AD) between the Warring States period and the Qin-Han period. The *Huang Di New Jing* is thought to be the summation of Chinese medical knowledge during the Han dynasty. In the first 81 sections of the book, the *Su Wen* ("Basic Questions"), the Yellow Emperor asks a series of questions of Qi Bo, a TCM practitioner, who explains the answers. The second 81 sections, the *Ling Shu* ("Spiritual Pivot"), is comprised of the clinical application of the Basic Questions and includes the different types of acupuncture needles, the meridian pathways, and the treatment of various pathological issues. This book is still used today in the study of TCM and TEAM as a foundational textbook.

Modern TEAM uses acupuncture as one of its forms of treatment. Other types of treatment used on the outside of the body include specialized manual manipulation/massage techniques (tui na), moxibustion, cupping, and gua sha. (More on exactly what those methods are later.)

The TEAM system uses herbal medicines similarly to the way that conventional medicine uses pharmaceuticals. Herbal medicines might be delivered internally by swallowing them as a tea, soup, powder, pill, or tincture. A person might inhale them like a nasal spray. They can also be delivered externally by placing them topically on the skin in the form of a poultice or patch.

TEAM places a strong emphasis on food as medicine, a phrase that has become popular these days but means something different in TEAM than it does on health-focused websites. The dietary recommendations given to you by a licensed acupuncturist are based on the energetic and physical properties of the foods and how they influence various organs in your body—not just your digestive system and their component macronutrients and micronutrients.

In TEAM, this includes methods of cooking, using herbs and spices, times of day appropriate for eating and for fasting, and other dietary choices. The line between herbal medicine and food medicine is very thin because many of the herbs are foods and vice versa. Cinnamon, ginger, and turmeric are all foods that are well-researched to have medicinal healing uses and are used in TEAM not only to flavor food but for specific medical purposes.

Exercise is an important component of TEAM. Tai Chi, also spelled "Taiji" or "Taijiquan," is a Chinese martial art that is often translated as "supreme ultimate" or "great extremes," reflecting its therapeutic mind-body foundations. Tai Chi is characterized by slow, flowing movements and a focus on meditative components including deep breathing and relaxation. You have likely seen pictures or videos of small groups of people practicing this fluid form of martial arts in settings like a park. There are many forms and styles of Tai Chi.

Another form of exercise called Qi Gong (also spelled "Qigong" or "Chi Kung") similarly involves coordinated body posture and movement, breathing, and meditation. The term is often translated as "life energy cultivation" or "cultivating energy." It involves slow, gentle movements, deep rhythmic breathing, and focused meditation to cultivate and balance Qi. Qi Gong can be done by a practitioner on a patient or can be used by a patient on themselves. Like Tai Chi, different styles and forms of Qi Gong exist, each with its specific movements, breathing patterns, and philosophical underpinnings. While some forms are more focused on health and relaxation, others are incorporated into martial arts training.

Licensed acupuncturists are the only kind of providers who are extensively trained in the use of all of these techniques as a part of their formal education. They may use some or all of these healing methods as a part of your treatment.

## SEE ALSO

- "What other kinds of things can an acupuncturist do?" *pg 145*
- "What is the history of acupuncture in the West?" *pg 159*
- "How does the thought theory of acupuncture differ from conventional medicine?" *pg 163*
- "Why does the acupuncturist want to see my tongue and feel my wrists?" *pg 130*

## Q. What are Yin and Yang?

Health in TEAM is based on the concept of balance. The Taiji symbol below—on its most basic level—represents that balance, and the two components that make up the balance are Yin and Yang.

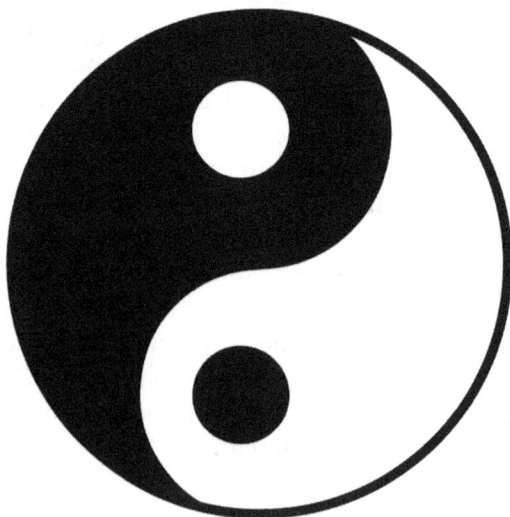

Yin is the darker of the two halves of the image and represents, among many other descriptors, darkness, cold, rest, recovery, heaviness, interior, descending, and stasis. Yang is the lighter part of the image and represents light, heat, activity, growth, lightness, exterior, rising, and movement. In order to be healthy, Yin activities like rest and recuperation (generally parasympathetic nervous system functions) must be balanced with Yang activity and movement (generally sympathetic nervous system functions).

Yin and Yang are two sides of the same coin. We better understand the concept of "full" because there is "empty." We know what "tall" is because we can compare it to "short." We can conceptualize "wide" because we also see "narrow." Even our earliest definitions of ourselves and our society are often based on these either-or characteristics (child or adult, left-handed or right-handed, big family or small family, rural or urban neighborhood), and childhood vocabulary develops around games of opposites. The whole of the world can be divided in this way and viewed in pairs. Yin and Yang help us to define and understand our world through their contrast.

### Four Characteristics of Yin and Yang

To dive a little deeper, there are 4 principle characteristics of Yin and Yang. The first teaches that because they are **interdependent** and define each other, one cannot exist without the other. We understand darkness because we contrast it to light. If we had darkness all the time, there would be no Yin-Yang pairing in the 24-hour cycle. The definition of Yin depends on there being a Yang contrast.

Yin and Yang are also in **opposition** to each other. They control and press against each other. You can visualize this by thinking about the weather patterns. The Yin time of the year is the cold winter. The Yang time of the year is the hot summer. In the fall and spring, Yin and Yang are transitioning one into the other, so some days are more Yang and hot and others are more Yin and cool. Hot Yang air and cold Yin air press against each other to create wind and weather patterns like thunderstorms and snow. Our choices about what we want to do in response to Yin and Yang are also in opposition to each other. We respond to cool Yin weather by doing quiet Yin activities like snuggling on the couch with a good book. In the warm Yang weather, we like to be outside running around and doing active, Yang things.

There is always a seed (represented by the dot in the image above) of one inside the other: within Yin you will find Yang and within Yang you will find Yin. They transform into each other. **Inter-transformation** is the third principle. We see this when a Yang fever turns to Yin chills and then back to a Yang fever.

As Yin swells and becomes bigger and more powerful, it diminishes Yang and vice versa, which is the principle of **mutual consumption**. I think this is the most challenging concept, but it builds on the idea of inter-transformation. Because they can transform into each other, when you decrease Yin, you decrease Yang. You might think about mutual consumption like a Yang fire blazing on Yin wood. The more the Yang fire burns, the more Yin wood it consumes. Conversely, the more Yin wood you put on the fire, the stronger the Yang fire grows. Eventually both the Yang and the Yin are consumed—the fire dies when there is no more wood.

### Yin and Yang in the Human Body

Yin is more strongly associated with the physical body—the blood ("Xue"), the body fluids ("Jin Ye") like saliva and tears, and the physicality of our bodies. Yin is the solid parts of you—the parts you can touch and the more substantive, solid organs. It is associated with stereotypically female bodies and functions such as menstruation (losing blood), creating new human bodies (babies) out of the mother's body, and receiving (the egg waiting for the sperm). The female genitalia are oriented into the body (Yin) and receive. The womb is deep inside the pelvic bowl. The egg waits for the sperm to arrive. The egg does not effort in this process. The egg just drifts along the fallopian tube in a very passive, relaxed Yin way and waits for the sperm to swim (Yang) to it and compete (Yang) for the opportunity to unite with it.

Yang is the energy of the body and manifests in the body as "Qi." Yang is the action part of you and describes whether or not you have lots of energy and are bouncing off the walls or have lower energy and prefer to be still. Yang organs are generally hollow and use lots of active, squeezing energy to move fluids or solids through them. Yang is associated with stereotypically male bodies and functions, many of which are action-oriented and outward-facing. The most obvious of these is the male genitalia, which are on the outside Yang part of the body and project outward during copulation and ejaculation. The sperm expends tremendous energy to travel a long distance to find the egg. You need Yin and Yang energies to be equal and balanced in order to form a new human being.

Once you begin to look around you and play the childhood game of "opposites," you will begin to notice the Yin and Yang aspects of the objects, animals, people, etc. of your surroundings and your community.

## SEE ALSO

- "What is Qi?" *pg 20*
- "How many acupuncture points are there?" *pg 66*
- "How does the thought theory of acupuncture differ from conventional medicine?" *pg 163*

## Q. What is Qi?

For the sake of clarity for the reader, I have chosen to use the Chinese term "Qi" throughout this book. An alternative spelling for "Qi" is "Chi," and both are pronounced "chee." The equivalent term in Japanese is "Ki" and in Korean is "Gi."

Qi is...energy. I dislike the term "energy" because it has been co-opted to mean that energetic things are woo-woo, and "energy" is therefore commonly dismissed in scientific circles. However, energy is a very important concept in science too. Physics, chemistry, biology, and biochemistry all understand energy as a driver of making things happen. I am going to do my best to walk the line for you between woo-woo energy and science energy as I explain Qi.

Qi is energy in the sense of having enough energy to do the things you want to do in your life. It is energy in the sense of the metabolism of your body being sufficient to sustain your life and vitality. It is energy in the sense of the glow around you when you have had a good night's sleep and feel recharged and ready for the day. It is energy in the sense that your stomach's energy should go down (digestion) and not up (vomiting or reflux/heartburn). It is the energy of a positive or negative emotional state. Qi is also the difference between life and death.

As an MD, I have walked into a patient's hospital room to find that they have passed away and seen people die in front of me in the trauma bay or operating room. Putting aside all of the emotions around that for a moment, there is something about the person's body that is a bit deflated when they die. It's true that their chest is not rising and falling anymore, but that is not it. As best I can describe it, it is something in their body shape and their skin. They are sunken. The energy that was holding the body in its living shape is gone.

From a TEAM perspective, the component that is missing after they have died is their Qi. The Yin of their physical body is still there, but the Yang (Qi) has departed. Their energy is gone. There are many religious terms for this kind of Qi—soul, spirit, essence, consciousness, etc.—but they mean similar things. There is a component of the person's aliveness that is now not there anymore. That life vitality is Yang Qi. When the Yang energy separates from the Yin physical body, the person dies.

The Chinese written language (Hanzi) is logographic. The Japanese Kanji and Korean Hanja are also logographic. This means that the lines create images that represent words or parts of words. When you analyze the components of the characters, the picture of the word gives you a little story about the word and its meaning. Here is the word for "Qi."

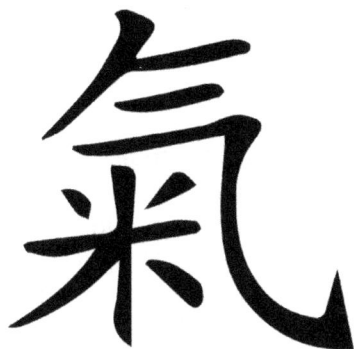

氣

There are two primary components of this character of "Qi." On the top, the horizontal lines represent steam coming out from underneath the lid of a pot. This is like a person's steamy, warm, Yang breath exhaling into the air on a cold, Yin day. On the bottom, the four small, diagonal lines around the "+" are representative of grains of rice. To cook the rice and make Qi that gives your body energy, it takes an appropriate amount of Yin water and Yang fire.

To go a little deeper into nutrition science, rice is comprised of simple sugars like glucose. We breathe in oxygen and breathe out carbon dioxide and water. So the ancient image of Qi is made up of the breath/steam plus glucose/rice combining to make energy.

In conventional medicine, we know about a molecule called adenosine triphosphate (ATP). This molecule is the "battery" of the cells: we put biochemical energy into ATP and then use the stored battery energy of ATP to power the biochemistry of life.

The way that we make ATP is by breaking down glucose (sugar) into pyruvate and running it through a series of steps in the Citric Acid Cycle to make high energy electrons. Those high energy electrons go into the Electron Transport Chain that push ADP (adenosine di-phosphate) to bind with phosphate to make ATP. Then those electrons are dumped onto oxygen ($O_2$ gas), they make water ($H_2O$) and carbon dioxide ($CO_2$ gas).

So the biochemical steps needed to make the energy molecule of ATP are: we inhale oxygen and eat glucose, process the glucose into ATP, and exhale the carbon dioxide mixed with water—the steam of our breath as we exhale. The TEAM steps needed to make Qi energy are inhaling and exhaling the breath combined with the consumption of simple carbohydrates like rice. I think it's amazing that the TEAM concept of Qi energy is largely the same as the conventional understanding of ATP energy—but from thousands of years before there were microscopes and the concepts of biochemistry and electrons!

When acupuncturists recommend foods, they are helping you make Qi. When they prescribe herbs, they are supporting the creation and movement and direction of your Qi. When they place acupuncture needles, they are manipulating, releasing, and guiding your Qi. Qi is a component of what we are feeling in your pulses and seeing on your tongue. Qi is the sensation of warmth or a pleasant ache ("de Qi" sensation) that you feel when the acupuncture needles are in place. Qi makes sure you move your bowels in the morning, retreats to let you fall asleep at night, and keeps your muscles engaged and functioning.

But of course, Qi has to be balanced with its counterpart, Xue. Yang/Qi invigorates and moves with the Yin/Xue Blood. Yin/Xue Blood moistens and nourishes the Yang/Qi. Yin and Yang, Xue and Qi, Blood and Energy sustain and balance each other. It is the acupuncturist's work—with your food choices and lifestyle choices—to support or control these components of your anatomy and physiology and bring your Yin body and Yang energy into balance with the intention of keeping you healthy and maintaining your longevity.

## SEE ALSO

- "What is Traditional East Asian Medicine (TEAM)?" *pg 13*
- "What are Yin and Yang?" *pg 16*
- "Why does the acupuncturist want to see my tongue and feel my wrists?" *pg 130*
- "Do the needles hurt?" *pg 114*

## Q. What is Five Element Theory?

Five Element Theory (FET) (also called "Five Phase Theory") is just one way of putting the body together in TEAM. While explaining how acupuncture works to medical students and to patients over the years, I have found that this theory seems to make the most sense to our western brains. Because of this, I am including only FET in this book and respectfully refer the reader to the References section for information on other foundational approaches to TEAM.

As with all of the theories in TEAM, FET is based on fastidious observation of the natural world and how humans fit into—and reflect—that naturalism. The five elements themselves are, unsurprisingly, named for natural substances: Earth, Metal, Water, Wood, and Fire. Each element is associated with Yin and Yang organs in the body, meridians, tissue types, flavors, sensory organs, times of the day, seasons of the year, and weather patterns. Among other things, the elements are also used to describe emotional states and tendencies toward one health problem or another. In this way, FET is predictive of the kinds of pathology a person will develop when they do not consistently make the lifestyle and dietary choices needed to keep themselves in balance. Likewise, when a person is performing tasks strongly associated with each element, they will have a tendency to develop the health problems associated with that element. More on that a bit later in the book. Let's first spend some time with the relationships of the elements to each other.

While each element relates to all the other elements, the way that they relate is very specific. Going around the outside, clockwise circle, the elements support each other by "generating" the element that comes after them. Each element likewise receives support from the one before. For example, Fire supports Earth, and Earth supports Metal. This means that in order to be healthy, the support that Earth receives from Fire must be equal to the degree that Earth is asked to support Metal. If Metal becomes too demanding, Earth can't support it properly and demands more from Fire. If Fire doesn't have enough to give, Earth becomes depleted.

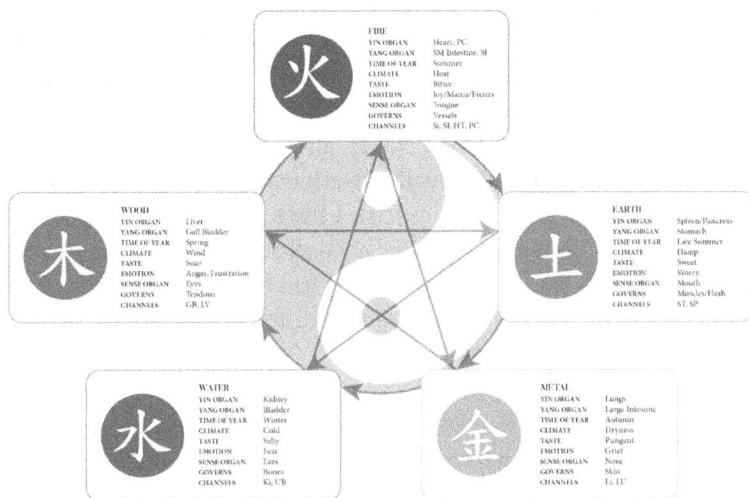

| FIRE | |
| --- | --- |
| YIN ORGAN | Heart, PC |
| YANG ORGAN | SM Intestine, SI |
| TIME OF YEAR | Summer |
| CLIMATE | Heat |
| TASTE | Bitter |
| EMOTION | Joy/Mania/Frenzy |
| SENSE ORGAN | Tongue |
| GOVERNS | Vessels |
| CHANNELS | Si, SI, HT, PC |

| WOOD | |
| --- | --- |
| YIN ORGAN | Liver |
| YANG ORGAN | Gall Bladder |
| TIME OF YEAR | Spring |
| CLIMATE | Wind |
| TASTE | Sour |
| EMOTION | Anger, Frustration |
| SENSE ORGAN | Eyes |
| GOVERNS | Tendons |
| CHANNELS | GB, LV |

| EARTH | |
| --- | --- |
| YIN ORGAN | Spleen/Pancreas |
| YANG ORGAN | Stomach |
| TIME OF YEAR | Late Summer |
| CLIMATE | Damp |
| TASTE | Sweet |
| EMOTION | Worry |
| SENSE ORGAN | Mouth |
| GOVERNS | Muscles/Flesh |
| CHANNELS | ST, SP |

| WATER | |
| --- | --- |
| YIN ORGAN | Kidney |
| YANG ORGAN | Bladder |
| TIME OF YEAR | Winter |
| CLIMATE | Cold |
| TASTE | Salty |
| EMOTION | Fear |
| SENSE ORGAN | Ears |
| GOVERNS | Bones |
| CHANNELS | Ki, UB |

| METAL | |
| --- | --- |
| YIN ORGAN | Lungs |
| YANG ORGAN | Large Intestine |
| TIME OF YEAR | Autumn |
| CLIMATE | Dryness |
| TASTE | Pungent |
| EMOTION | Grief |
| SENSE ORGAN | Nose |
| GOVERNS | Skin |
| CHANNELS | Li, LU |

The other way that the elements relate to each other is represented by the lines that form the star: the "controlling" cycle. Fire keeps Metal in check and prevents it from getting too big for its britches. Metal controls Wood. Wood controls Earth and so on. If Wood is kind of a jerk and "over controls" Earth, Earth gets depleted. Earth might also "rebel" and give the middle finger to Wood to get it to back off and stop being such a bully. You can see that each element is like a child in the sandbox: they can be supportive and generous, but they can also be controlling or rebellious at a moment's notice.

These supporting and controlling relationships extend to all aspects of the element. For example, bitter kale chips taste much better with sour vinegar and salty salt. (There is a reason there are five spices in Chinese Five Spice blend.) If we think about the emotional aspects of the elements, Wood is decisive and controls Earth's proclivity to be pensive and introspective. From a physical perspective, Fire generates Earth/earth (soil) when it burns up Wood/wood. From a tissue type perspective, the Wood tendons/ligaments are supported by the Water bones.

As a medical doctor, I can think about your lungs in relative isolation and maybe even send you to a Pulmonologist who will focus almost entirely on your lungs. But in TEAM, we don't think in isolated systems. You can see that Earth supports Metal, and Metal supports Water. Fire controls Metal, and Metal controls Wood. In this way, each organ has a specific relationship to every other organ in the system. As an acupuncturist, I **have** to think about you as a whole person. I **have** to consider how all the other organs in your body are interacting with your Lungs to create the problems with your breathing. This is a foundational difference between conventional medicine and TEAM.

Conventional medicine tends to take each body system and specialize and super specialize and look at smaller and smaller aspects of a person to find the one specific diagnosis that explains that headache you have or the reason why your white blood cell count is high. It's a reductionist form of medicine. It's great for figuring out very specific issues. TEAM tends to look at all of those smaller pieces as symptoms of a larger root cause and then treat the root, anticipating that the interrelated branches will all improve as the root becomes healthier. It's a holistic form of medicine. It's great for looking at the big picture. Both are helpful, depending on your healthcare needs, but they are opposite ways of thinking and opposite approaches to care.

With the level of medical information we now know, conventional doctors have to know too many details about too many details to really think holistically, in my opinion. It is just asking too much of them. They aren't allowed time to think outside of their specialty anymore—it all has to be immediately clinically relevant because anything more is just too exhausting and overwhelming. But I digress...

When I see patients for the first time in clinic, they often come with a long list of problems. They are so relieved to learn that all of their issues can be explained in the context of these TEAM Five

Element relationships. They don't really have a long list of unrelated issues: they just have an imbalanced system. Once we get the individual elements to work together harmoniously by treating the root cause of their issues—once the generating and controlling cycles come back into balance—they are amazed at how much better they feel and how quickly seemingly insurmountable issues begin to resolve.

This, my friend, is the true power of TEAM. It sees people as a whole. It treats people as a whole. It seeks relationships between the systems, the emotions, the food, the activity level, and the tissues. It recognizes that you are an individual who has inherited a set of Jing patterns from your parents and has had experiences and made lifestyle choices that have brought you to this place in your health journey with these health concerns. Without judgment, it then helps you unpack those elemental relationships and teaches you to tweak your choices so that they are in alignment with what you want your health to be. It shows us that, while aging is inevitable, maintaining health as best we can is simply a matter of balance. By understanding our proclivities to support or control or rebel against one element or another, we can find that balance.

## SEE ALSO

- "What does the Earth/Metal/Water/Wood/Fire Element (Phase) represent?" *pgs 23-46*
- "What does the Water Element represent?" pg 33 *(for a definition of "Jing.")*
- "Why are emotions so important in Traditional East Asian Medicine?" *pg 46*
- "How does the thought theory of acupuncture differ from conventional medicine?" *pg 163*

- "How does an acupuncturist formulate a diagnosis and treatment plan?" *pg 56*
- "Why does the acupuncturist want to see my tongue and feel my wrists?" *pg 130*

## Q. What does the Earth Element represent?

If you skipped to this question without reading "What is Five Element Theory?" I suggest that you go back and read that one first before proceeding with each of the individual elements.

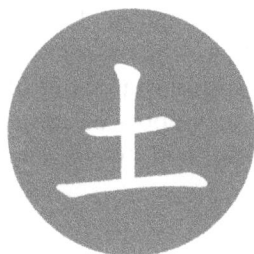

### EARTH

| | |
|---|---|
| YIN ORGAN | Spleen/Pancreas |
| YANG ORGAN | Stomach |
| TIME OF YEAR | Late Summer |
| CLIMATE | Damp |
| TASTE | Sweet |
| EMOTION | Worry |
| SENSE ORGAN | Mouth |
| GOVERNS | Muscles/Flesh |
| CHANNELS | ST, SP |

The Earth element is associated with the beginnings of the digestive process and how we create the flesh of ourselves from the fruits of the earth. It is linked to the Spleen (which some scholars would assert is more correctly translated as the Spleen/Pancreas) and Stomach organs and meridians, the flesh, the mouth, and the sweet flavor. Earth people tend to be particularly sensitive to damp, humid weather—the kind of weather that is common in the late summer season. They prefer to wake up, exercise, go to bed, etc. at

the same time each day and do best when they stick to a schedule. Earth people tend to feel grounded when they have a routine, and they develop habits easily.

People with a lot of Earth proclivities have a tendency to chew on their thoughts. On the healthy end of the spectrum, they tend to be pensive and introspective. When they are less balanced, they tend to worry or overthink things. In American colloquialisms, we similarly connect thinking with eating. For example, when we want to consider something carefully, we might say, "I will chew on that," meaning "I will think on that." We say "that's food for thought." We even use the word "ruminate" to mean we will turn over our thoughts the same way that cows (ruminants) chew their cud.

The sweet flavor is associated with Earth. I find it interesting that culinary medical science backs up this observation. When we are worried or anxious, we like the pleasant chemical messengers that eating a sweet treat creates in our body. When we are studying and using our minds intensely to figure out a problem, our brains want simple carbohydrates—sweets. When was the last time you were craving celery when you were staying up all night studying for a test? There are all-night cookie delivery services located near college campuses for a reason.

We are all aware that eating sweets can make us more fleshy (think paintings by Botacelli—people with "meat on their bones"), which is the tissue type associated with the Earth element. Earth-type people tend to be naturally more fleshy than other elemental types, but people gravitate (see what I did there?) to Earth types because they are naturally warm, generous, and supportive of others. They remember everyone's birthday and are dependable. They benevolently open the circle to hear everyone's side and include everyone's opinions. If you are in need of some genuine caring and an affectionate hug, someone to help resolve a dispute, or a guide in building compassion for yourself or others, seek out an Earth person.

### SEE ALSO

- "What is Five Element Theory?" *pg 23*
- "What does the Earth/Metal/Water/Wood/Fire Element (Phase) represent?" *pgs 23-46*
- "Why are emotions so important in Traditional East Asian Medicine?" *pg 46*
- "What are acupuncture channels or meridians? What are acupoints?" *pg 65*
- "Why does the acupuncturist want to see my tongue and feel my wrists?" *pg 130*

## Q. What does the Metal Element represent?

If you skipped to this question without reading "What is Five Element Theory?" I suggest that you go back and read that one first before proceeding with each of the individual elements.

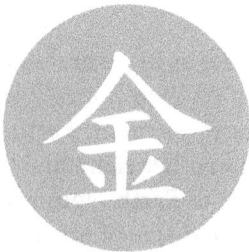

| METAL | |
|---|---|
| YIN ORGAN | Lungs |
| YANG ORGAN | Large Intestine |
| TIME OF YEAR | Autumn |
| CLIMATE | Dryness |
| TASTE | Pungent |
| EMOTION | Grief |
| SENSE ORGAN | Nose |
| GOVERNS | Skin |
| CHANNELS | Li, LU |

The Metal element is our armor. It is how we protect ourselves from the outside world. As such, it goes with the tissue type of the skin—the physical border that differentiates our human form from the outside world. Metal organs and channels are the Lungs and Large Intestine (or Colon). That might sound like a goofy pairing, but the Lungs and Large Intestine are the most external of the internal organs. They define our borders.

The Metal organs and tissues protect us from outside invaders by being large repositories of immune system cells and major routes of communication between the endocrine, immune, and neurological systems in our bodies. Since TEAM is thousands of years older than microscopes and the concept of cells, the early TEAM texts admittedly don't specifically say anything about an immune system. (The immune system hadn't been invented/discovered yet.) However, the concept of defending yourself from outside invasion is absolutely discussed in the ancient textbooks as being associated with the Metal system. So Metal = protection = immune function, according to our modern understanding.

As I mentioned, the Lungs and Large Intestine are the organs closest to the outside and exchange air with the atmosphere and waste with the earth (Earth supports Metal). With the Lungs, we can choose how to interface with the world—or not. The Lungs are also the only organs that works without our having to think about it, but that we can control with our thoughts. In other words, we breathe automatically, but we also have the power to take a deep breath and hold it. The breath is also the first way that we define life: we take our first and last breath.

The Large Intestine releases waste back to the Earth to be recycled. It also brings back in water and other organic molecules for recycling in the body. The microbiome is a complex ecosystem of viruses, yeasts, bacteria (and other heebee jeebies you don't want to think about in the night) that live in us and on us. One of the places that we rely most heavily on the functions of the microbiome is in our large intestine. The microbiome interacts with our immune system and our nervous system. If the ecosystem microbiome is not healthy and balanced, we are not healthy and balanced either.

The plants change carbon dioxide into oxygen and give it back to us, forming a cycle built on letting go of each breath and the trust that the next inhale will provide us with what we need. Letting go of something or someone we cared for is sad. As such, grief and sadness are the emotions associated with Metal. Metal helps us to honor the passage of time, and we do that by acknowledging that life is short. When we grieve, we are honoring time and the brevity of the stages or span of life within it. Autumn, the time of year when the plants have to let go of their leaves and the world dies a little death as it transitions into Winter, is the time of year associated with Metal.

Metal organs and tissues (skin) need a little moisture in their lives and don't do well with Dryness. The Lungs respond to dry weather or climate with a dry persistent cough. One of the Large Intestine's jobs is to reabsorb water. If we are very dehydrated, the stool becomes too dry and can become difficult or painful to pass. The Autumn weather begins to be more dry, and our immune systems are challenged with infections that cause upper respiratory infections (in our nose and lungs) or infections in the digestive system (that result in diarrhea or constipation).

The Metal organs are associated with boundaries such as defining inside vs outside, inhale vs exhale, food vs waste, me (inside my skin) and not me (outside my skin), me (not an invading pathogen) vs not me (invading pathogen that the immune system attacks). Metal people really love their boundaries. They like to know what time you're going to arrive and when you will leave. They love rules, order, law, definitions, and precision. They don't understand why other people feel it is OK to bend or break the rules and are often incredulous that others would even think of such a thing. The "tattle tale" in your elementary school class was almost certainly a Metal child. Because they make distinctions easily, Metal people have an excellent moral compass and memorize things easily. They are tidy, organized and prepared. If you are looking for a fair judge who can see both sides of an issue and still come to a decisive conclusion or for a person who will help you create a system that is unbiased and logical with clear expectations and deadlines for everyone, seek out a Metal person.

---

### SEE ALSO

- "What is Five Element Theory?" *pg 23*
- "What does the Earth/Metal/Water/Wood/Fire Element (Phase) represent?" *pgs 23-46*
- "Why are emotions so important in Traditional East Asian Medicine?" *pg 46*
- "What are acupuncture channels or meridians? What are acupoints?" *pg 65*
- "Why does the acupuncturist want to see my tongue and feel my wrists?" *pg 130*

---

## Q. What does the Water Element represent?

If you skipped to this question without reading "What is Five Element Theory?" I suggest that you go back and read that one first before proceeding with each of the individual elements.

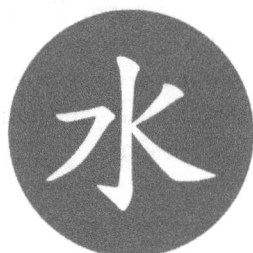

**WATER**

| | |
|---|---|
| YIN ORGAN | Kidney |
| YANG ORGAN | Bladder |
| TIME OF YEAR | Winter |
| CLIMATE | Cold |
| TASTE | Salty |
| EMOTION | Fear |
| SENSE ORGAN | Ears |
| GOVERNS | Bones |
| CHANNELS | Ki, UB |

The food that we eat (Earth) and the air that we breathe (Metal) together form what we have to work with each day. I like to say Earth + Metal = our checking account. We try not to overdraft our checking account, but in times of great stress (death of a loved one, long standing work stress, chronic insomnia, physical or emotional trauma), we need to dip into a savings account. That savings account is the Water element.

Water...you probably guessed...goes with the Kidneys and Urinary Bladder and is associated with our "genetic" proclivities. I put this in quotation marks because the genetics (family history) that are important for this or that problem in conventional medicine is very limited. We medical doctors want to know about cholesterol and diabetes and heart problems in the family, but we don't ask about whether there is a family history of low back pain or headaches or abdominal bloating. We just don't think it is relevant.

But in TEAM, you inherit some "Jing" from Dad and some "Jing" from Mom. (Jing is the reproductive Yin and Yang that forms the vital force responsible for creating a new human. When Jing is depleted, the vital force is exhausted, the person's Yin and Yang separate, and they die.) Those two parental Jing components combine together to make the first Kidney that is you. Then that initial Kidney splits into two Kidneys. One is more associated with Yin physical characteristics: we look like Mom and Dad or have pro-clivities to have XYZ health problems like Mom and Dad do (as in "everyone has a bad heart in our family" or "the Jones family gut problems"). The other Kidney is more associated with Yang functions. For example, we might have similar behaviors, likes/dislikes, or energy levels to one or both of our parents. You can see that Jing is kinda like the conventional medical concept of characteristics and traits passing from parents to offspring through the genes, but it is also the vital force that is you as a separate being when you are engendered from that Jing. It is the force of your life.

Water is associated with the adrenal glands, the gonads (ovaries and testes), and brain—strange connections to our western ways of thinking. But embryologically, the kidneys and the brain begin to form right around the same time and are closely related to each other. Likewise, when you are developing in the womb, the adrenals, kidneys and gonads are right on top of each other. As you elongate from a short tube of cells into a longer, worm-like shape, the gonads descend down into your pelvis (and out of your pelvis if you are male), and the adrenal glands sit like little pyramids on top of the kidneys. The Water tissue type is the bones, and the brain can be considered to be a specialized kind of tissue housed (like marrow) in the bone.

Fear and fright are the emotions associated with the Water element. When we get startled, we might lose control of our urine and our heart might stop for a moment, dying a tiny—albeit impermanent—death. We even say "you scared the life out of me." Living a life that is full of stress and fear tends to prematurely age people. Around age 40, it becomes obvious whether or not someone has had a life in which they were able to sustain their needs with just their Earth and Metal checking account or if they have had to dip into their Water savings account regularly.

Water people don't necessarily tend to look older in the face, but they do tend to go gray before their peers or have "old people problems" like low back pain or knee issues at a younger age. This is because, as we age, our Water savings account becomes depleted, and people who have a lot of Water tendencies don't have as much reserve as other element types.

As a part of normal aging, we lose our hearing (the ears are the orifice for the Kidney system). We lose our reproductive abilities to pass on our genes/Jing to the next generation. (Because Yin/women menstruate and lose so much blood/Blood/Yin over their lifetimes, they lose this ability before Yang/men do and often suffer with Yang hot flashes). Our bones might become brittle and the mind—housed in the bone of the skull—might not work as well as it used to. We might struggle with kidney stones (from salt imbalances), blood pressure control (from the kidneys not regulating salt and water balance as well), or bladder control (from Qi weakness in the Yang Urinary Bladder). As we age, we lose Yang heat. We need more clothes and become more sensitive to cold. We can't move as fast because we have less Yang Qi.

These aging processes are all parts of moving into the Winter of our lives. Winter is also the time of "being the seed" and envisioning the potential of what a person might become. The darkness of the winter solstice causes us to reflect, be still, and create quiet peacefulness around us. Without that time of introspection, we would never develop wisdom or be able to change the direction of our lives in the Spring.

Water is an easygoing element. It tends to conform to whatever vessel holds it, and Water people are similarly laissez faire, easygoing, contented kind of people. They let problems roll off of them with relative ease—like "water off a duck's back." Even though they go grey or lose their hair at an early age—making them appear older than they actually are—they likewise tend to be wise and insightful beyond their years, which gives them a strong sense of self worth. Water people are loyal and courageous friends. They love to consider things deeply, play mentally challenging games, and banter with others about complicated abstract concepts. Philosophers and poets are often Water people. If you are looking for someone who will rumble with you about complicated problems, not get sucked in by any unfounded assertions, and provide you with sage advice, look for a Water person.

## SEE ALSO

- "What is Five Element Theory?" *pg 23*
- "What does the Earth/Metal/Water/Wood/Fire Element (Phase) represent?" *pgs 23-46*
- "Why are emotions so important in Traditional East Asian Medicine?" *pg 46*
- "What are acupuncture channels or meridians? What are acupoints?" *pg 65*
- "Why does the acupuncturist want to see my tongue and feel my wrists?" *pg 130*

## Q. What does the Wood Element represent?

If you skipped to this question without reading "What is Five Element Theory?" I suggest that you go back and read that one first before proceeding with each of the individual elements.

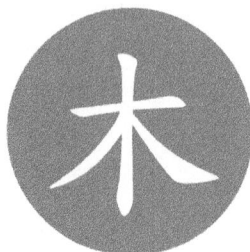

**WOOD**

| | |
|---|---|
| YIN ORGAN | Liver |
| YANG ORGAN | Gall Bladder |
| TIME OF YEAR | Spring |
| CLIMATE | Wind |
| TASTE | Sour |
| EMOTION | Anger, Frustration |
| SENSE ORGAN | Eyes |
| GOVERNS | Tendons |
| CHANNELS | GB, LV |

Wood is associated with the Liver and Gallbladder. The Liver is the Yin organ of the pair and as such has a pretty tricky job description. On the one hand, it is a squishy, blood-filled organ—which you can attest to if you've ever seen one in the grocery store. One of Liver's jobs is to store and hold Blood. But the other job is to regulate and smooth the flow of Qi in the body. So if Blood (Yin) and Qi (Yang) are supposed to circulate together, how can you possibly hold one and move the other? Pretty challenging. So the emotion that goes with the Wood system is frustration, which I'm going to spend a bit of extra time talking with you about.

Frustration is considered to be a "bad" emotion in our culture. But the beauty of frustration is that it drives change. If we didn't get frustrated, we would never leave our parent's house. Because they drive us crazy, we move out. We leave our jobs because we are frustrated. We get a new degree because we are frustrated. We look for other life partners or other friends because we are frustrated with our current situation. Frustration is a powerful, amazing emotion and is just the push we need to imagine something better for ourselves and go out and find it. Change is big and scary, but frustration eventually pushes us to change anyway.

We even see frustration driving change in nature. The Spring is the time of new shoots coming up out of the ground because they are dissatisfied with their current seed-like state and envision something bigger and better for themselves. They push all of the Earthy soil (Wood controls Earth) out of the way so that they can extend themselves into the Wind and grow.

Wood is represented by bamboo—a decidedly goal-oriented plant. If you put an obstacle on top of bamboo, it will just go around the obstacle and go back to what it was doing. Potential source of frustration resolved. But if we can't get out from under our frustration, it goes one of two ways, generally. We get angry and start yelling and screaming at people in traffic, on the elevator, or at home. Or we become so frustrated because every time we turn around to try to make a change the door just keeps getting slammed in our face, so why bother? That is depression and hopelessness. Instead of outward screaming angry frustration, this depressed frustration tends to be turned inward. We start to tell ourselves we are worthless, and we can't make good decisions.

When you are raised in a competitive culture that tells you that you must be #1 in everything at all times—including a perfect house, car, significant other, kid(s), dog, fingernails, yard, Christmas decorations, shoes, mustache, etc.—it is very difficult to not feel frustrated. We are not raised to prioritize satisfaction with what we have over desire for "more," "new," and "better." So we have a culture of chronically frustrated, angry, depressed people.

How do we combat frustration? With exercise. Yes, seriously. The Liver needs to be let out to run around the yard on a regular basis. You already know that exercise is not optional for you if you are a Wood person. Similarly, if you are frustrated, you might want to kick box, break some plates, throw an ax against the wall, or have a pillow fight. That Liver energy needs to MOVE before the anger erupts. Wood people should also avoid the heating effects of alcohol, which burns up the Yin of the Liver and makes them more frustrated/angry/depressed. But this is often the opposite of what they do because alcohol initially dulls the Liver and tricks the Woody person into thinking they are more relaxed.

The tissue type associated with the Wood element is the connective tissue—the tendons, ligaments and fascia. Connection is in some ways the opposite of frustration, and connective tissue allows us to bend and sway without breaking in the changing Winds of life. When Liver people are healthy, they are able to roll with the punches and get up again easily when knocked down. The tendons and ligaments need to be kept hydrated with moisturizing Yin Blood. When they dry out from Liver Heat, they tend to rip and tear.

In women, there is an added connection between the Liver and the Uterus. The old Yin Blood goes into the Uterus to be extruded from the body when a woman menstruates. This happens 2-3 days before the menstrual bleeding begins and leaves the body with a little bit less Yin cooling the Yang Qi. This is the TEAM explanation for why women have premenstrual headaches (hot Yang rising up and irritating the head, particularly behind or around the eyes), feel irritable (the Liver regulates the smoothness of emotions), and have painful symptoms like cramps, low back pain, and breast tenderness (stagnation of Qi in those areas that is exposed when there is a little less Yin Blood in circulation). Women tend to be "Yin deficient" as a consequence of losing all this Blood over their lifetime, which leads to hot flashes and night sweats when women enter menopause. These symptoms might be even stronger if a woman loses Yin by having babies (using the physicalness of her Yin to create the Yin of another human + the Yin Blood loss associated with pregnancy) or has bleeding issues from other causes like PCOS or fibroids.

I want to mention that what is "normal" in TEAM is that a woman's period comes regularly every 28 days. She bleeds for about 5 days without pain or clots or cramps and then the bleeding stops.

No spotting. No PMS. No irritability. No sleep disturbances. Her period just shows up, does its thing, and then stops, returning promptly at the same time each month. Everything else—all those other symptoms that conventional medicine considers a "normal" part of having a period and being genetically female—is not "normal" in TEAM. When you see a TEAM practitioner, this is something that is bread-and-butter acupuncture medicine. (You seriously don't have to live like that. Let an acupuncturist help you.)

Similarly, you don't have to live with the hot flashes and night sweats I mentioned above when your body decides to quit menstruating. I don't know how many women I've treated with those issues, but it is absolutely possible to just go from menstruating to not menstruating without the years and years of menopausal symptoms. On average, it takes me about 3-6 months to fix that problem and assist a woman's body in making the transition. You just don't have to suffer. That is not "normal" according to TEAM.

Men don't have a uterus, and so they don't have the benefit of cleaning out the old Yin Blood month to month. But they do have the benefit of not being chronically Yin deficient. Now back to the Wood system.

Wood people are decisive and visionary when they are healthy, but as we have discussed, they are depressed and angry when they are not. Exercise is critical for the mental health of Wood people in your life, and although they resist routine, they function better when they at least get up and go to bed at the same time each day. Wood people tend to have an easier time with change but also tend to not worry so much about details, rules, and regulations. (They need Metal people to help them with this—Metal controls Wood.) They tend to envision (Eyes) things as they should be and actively advocate for the transformation needed to create an idealistic, just society. If you need a goal-oriented, competitive, natural leader who works well under pressure, takes responsibility, and easily finds innovative solutions, look for a Wood person.

## SEE ALSO

- "What is Five Element Theory?" *pg 23*
- "What does the Earth/Metal/Water/Wood/Fire Element (Phase) represent?" *pgs 23-46*
- "Why are emotions so important in Traditional East Asian Medicine?" *pg 46*
- "What are acupuncture channels or meridians? What are acupoints?" *pg 65*
- "Why does the acupuncturist want to see my tongue and feel my wrists?" *pg 130*

## Q. What does the Fire Element represent?

If you skipped to this question without reading "What is Five Element Theory?" I suggest that you go back and read that one first before proceeding with each of the individual elements.

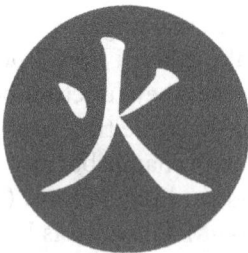

| FIRE | |
|---|---|
| YIN ORGAN | Heart, PC |
| YANG ORGAN | SM Intestine, SJ |
| TIME OF YEAR | Summer |
| CLIMATE | Heat |
| TASTE | Bitter |
| EMOTION | Joy/Mania/Frenzy |
| SENSE ORGAN | Tongue |
| GOVERNS | Vessels |
| CHANNELS | Si, SJ, HT, PC |

Finally, we come to Fire. You can see that Fire is comprised of two sets of organs. The Yin Heart and Pericardium (also translated as "Master of the Heart" or "Heart Protector"), and the Yang Small Intestine and San Jiao (Triple Heater or Triple Burner). We have two sets here because the Heart is the Emperor of the whole system. A normal person would never charge right in to see the Emperor. They would first go through a minister (and another minister and another minister) to get to the ruler. So to get to the Heart, a person must go through the Master of the Heart/Pericardium.

You can also think of the Heart as the sun and the Pericardium as the sunlight and heat emanating from the sun. The sun is much more powerful and intense, but it can be too much. It needs to be tempered so that it is not overwhelming. The Pericardium is the representative reflection of that power and intensity—just cooled down a little bit. Naturally, the season associated with Fire is the Yang hot middle of the summer, when the sun is the strongest and the light from the days is the longest.

More specifically, the heat of the Fire in the Yin Heart is necessary because we need the Heart to keep up the hot Yang function of beating every second of every minute of our lives. It is a Yin organ, but it has a lot of hot Yang energy. All that activity tends to cause the Heart to get overheated, and the Pericardium helps to cool the Heart just a little bit. (If the Pericardium fails in this job, the consequences are palpitations and strokes.)

Anatomically, this is very interesting. All the other organs in the body are just kind of hanging out there once you get below the skin and fascial layers. You can see all the belly organs right in front of you, for example, when you lift up the omental apron, a flap of tissue hanging down from the lower part of the stomach that looks like a 1950s housewife's apron. Similarly, if you open the chest, the lungs are right there beneath the connective pleural layers. But the heart has its own private chamber—the pericardium. The pericardial sac holds the heart in place and keeps it from flopping around as it is beating. It gives the heart room to move and offers a very thick, strong, protective barrier. This is unique. The heart is the only organ with a private room.

The Small Intestine has the job of taking in what is helpful and nutritive and letting go of what is not—passing waste along to the Large Intestine to be further processed and for recycling to happen. It separates things into what will become part of physical you and what will become waste. The Heart's job is similarly to take up experiences that will become part of you and let go of those that are not. You probably don't remember, for example, the number of seconds you spent at a stop sign this morning. But if a child suddenly rides out in front of you on their bike at that stop sign tomorrow, you will remember it ("take it to heart") and will be vigilant about that stop sign going forward. The Heart helps you to process all of the thoughts, emotions, experiences, and reactions that occur in your day and separate them into the relevant pile for remembering and the irrelevant pile that can be forgotten.

The Heart is strongly associated with your consciousness, personality, or "Shen." The Shen consciousness comes to rest in the Heart Blood at night. When it does this and the Heart Blood is cooling enough, you sleep. If there is not enough Yin Blood or the Yin Blood is too hot, sleep is disrupted. You might not be able to fall asleep. You might have vivid dreams or wake up often in the night. When that happens, you feel tired in the morning (Fire cannot support Earth) and struggle to get out of bed. You might feel more anxious and agitated during the day, leading you to bounce around from one thing to another, but unable to focus and concentrate on the issue at hand.

The Pericardium is paired with something for which we have no concept in conventional medicine. "San" in Chinese means "three" and a "Jiao" is a heater or burner. So San Jiao is the three centers of heat in the center of the body: the chest, abdomen, and pelvis. It also refers to the way that we regulate fluids (Yin) between those

Yang heat centers. Some scholars think the San Jiao also relates to the lymph system—how fluids get from the spaces outside the blood vessels (extravascular spaces) back into the blood vessels (vascular spaces)—but I struggle with this because the lymphatics also have a lot to do with immune function.

As a medical doctor, I have seen fluid in the belly due to liver failure build up so much that the fluid starts to leak into the chest cavity (ascites become a pleural effusion). I have seen similar fluid problems move between the abdomen and the pelvis. But this is not really something that conventional medicine focuses on as a concept. However, it is a very effective concept in TEAM. If you find that a person has a wet cough (chest), bloating and indigestion (abdomen), and struggles with urinary tract infections (pelvis), I would first evaluate and treat the San Jiao.

The emotion of the Fire element is joy, but this, as with all emotional states, is not "good" or "bad." Joy is the most common translation, but in my opinion, what is meant is "overjoyed." People who have imbalanced Fire are like Dolores Umbridge from the Harry Potter movies. They have a giggling way of talking and when they feel wronged, they tend toward bitterness. They tend to focus on self-satisfaction to bring themselves pleasure—these are manic or hypomanic types of behaviors. The heat in their system is just too hot, and it makes them feel frenzied.

When Fire people are in balance, they are the light that draws all the moths around them to the flame. They are vibrant, energetic, optimistic, and happy. They love to perform and bring joy to those around them, making even the most mundane of tasks playful and fun. Many actors and performers are Fire people, not only because they are passionate and creative, but also because they love to laugh and engage with new people easily. If you are feeling sad and need encouragement or compassion, seek out a Fire person. They will not be afraid to make you laugh at a funeral (Fire controls Metal), encourage you to trust your intuition, and relish every aspect of your life.

---

### SEE ALSO

- "What is Five Element Theory?" *pg 23*
- "What does the Earth/Metal/Water/Wood/Fire Element (Phase) represent?" *pgs 23-46*
- "Why are emotions so important in Traditional East Asian Medicine?" *pg 46*
- "What are acupuncture channels or meridians? What are acupoints?" *pg 65*
- "Why does the acupuncturist want to see my tongue and feel my wrists?" *pg 130*

---

## Q. Why are emotions so important in Traditional East Asian Medicine?

This is complicated. Because it's complicated, I'd like to start with where the word came from because I think it helps to focus our attention not just on the feeling of feelings, but on why we have them at all. The word "emotion" comes from the Latin "movere" meaning "to move." This is interesting first because it implies that emotions arise to move or direct us in one way or another. They are a driving force in our behavior. "Moving" also implies that emotions should move through us. They are not meant to stick around. Let's begin diving in by looking more closely at the idea that emotions motivate, move, and direct us.

Current biomedical research demonstrates that emotions arise in the body, not in the mind. In other words, they don't necessarily involve thoughts when they first show up. Thoughts come into play later on. Emotions are part of your reactions to the stimuli coming at you all the time in the context of the environment that you experience the stimuli. Heady stuff, I know. Let's break that down.

If you see something that looks scary out of the corner of your eye while you are walking home, this might cause your heart rate and breathing rate to speed up so that the blood can bring oxygen and nutrients to your big muscles. This allows you to use your big muscles to run away or to fight. The heart rate, breathing rate, and redistribution of blood are "autonomic" responses. (Notice the "auto" part of that word—like "automatic" and "auto-pilot.") Autonomic responses are intended to be automatic and to allow us to react to things in our environment quickly and with minimal conscious thought.

It would take too long to say to yourself, "Hmmm, I think that dog is growling at me. I have seen other dogs growl like that, and the outcome has not been good for the people they were growling at. Perhaps I should get ready to find something to defend myself with or to run away from this dog. And I might need a bit of adrenaline to get my heart beating harder and faster and increase my breathing. That adrenaline will also help to numb the pain that might happen if I stub my toe while I'm running away. Yeah, I should definitely get some adrenaline into my system even though it will make me feel shaky later on. Perhaps I should quit trying to digest the pizza I just ate for lunch and move my blood into my thigh muscles so I can get out of here. Oof, I have a little knot in my stomach now from the blood leaving my stomach and going into my thigh muscles, but that's OK. I'll come back to digest that food a little later ..."

That would take waaaaaay too long. You need to get out of harm's way by getting away from that dog immediately. Later on when you are safe, you might be able to think about the experience and realize that the dog wasn't actually growling at you but at another dog across the street. But in the moment, your body creates all of those automatic responses to keep you safe and alive—the most important drive as a human being. Your brain's rational abilities only show up later on after you are out of perceived danger.

You learn from your parents and others around you that the shaky feeling, knotted stomach, fast-beating heart, and rapid breathing in the context of sensing something that might cause you harm is part of a constellation of sensations that we call "fear" or "fright." You have all of the automatic physical and emotional reactions to the stimulus in fractions of a second. You don't have to think about being afraid to become afraid. Your body reacts to something with the potential to do harm and your autonomic changes and emotional response happen automatically. The naming and thoughtful processing and consideration of all of the stimuli happen later when we are not on auto-pilot.

We also learn to recognize that other autonomic responses have different emotion names and are similarly tied to context. A knot in the stomach in the context of seeing something scary is called "fear." A knot in the stomach in the context of getting ready to take an important test might be called "anxiety." A knot in the stomach when getting ready to kiss someone that we really like might be called "love." A knot in the stomach when we are getting to embark on a new adventure might be called "excitement."

What can be confusing when we are first experiencing this as children is that fear, anxiety, love, and excitement can all be associated with a knot in the stomach. They are similar autonomic "feelings" in the body. It is the context that defines the knot in the stomach as a different emotion, and we generally need adult help to figure out the differences. The mind (conscious thought) learns to distinguish the changes in the body in the context of what is going on when those changes happen and give those automatic, reactive, autonomic changes different emotional names. We learn to distinguish the feeling names based on subtlety between the various stomach knots and other autonomic changes and the context where we were when we had them.

As children, we need guidance to give these body sensations the names of the emotions we are feeling. When we have the name for what we are feeling, we can learn to communicate with those around us. We can tell a parent when we are afraid or anxious or excited, which means the parent can guide us in how to "deal" with the emotions we are experiencing. We learn how our emotions might guide our behavior when we experience those emotions. If we are not taught how to interpret the autonomic, automatic responses we are having from one moment to the other, we don't know how to make logical sense of our experiences. We fail to express ourselves accurately when talking about our emotions/reactions with others. We can't figure out how to respond with behaviors that avoid negative consequences.

If as a child you are only given a box of crayons that has eight emotional colors in it by the adults and peers around you, you only have eight emotional color names as you move into adulthood. You can only discuss the eight emotions that you can name and identify with adult friends, colleagues at work, and potential life partners. Your choices for expressing yourself are limited because you don't understand the nuances that might further widen the scope of your emotional range. Your life experiences are seen through the lens of only eight emotional options.

If people around you give you the names and subtle differences between additional emotional colors, you can start to name and distinguish green emotions from blue emotions and purple emotions. If you get even more emotional color names in your childhood, you now can talk about chartreuse, lavender, turquoise, and navy emotional colors. You learn to identify the subtle differences between what you are feeling in your body and the context you are feeling them because someone taught you where to look for those subtle signs.

The more vocabulary you have for yourself around the body information you are given when your stomach feels knotted and the context in which that is happening, the more your mind can help you to interpret the autonomic responses and help you to move along in your life. You can say to yourself, "I notice that my stomach is knotted, my hands are a little sweaty, and my heart rate is up...I might be feeling a little nervous right now, but I know that there is nothing to be concerned about. I am safe. Everything is going to be OK." You take a deep breath and head up to the lectern to give your presentation. Because you could identify it, name it, and take a breath to help you slow down your heart rate, your body responds to this self-coaching by calming down a little. You feel less nervous. You are better able to deliver your lecture because you have the appropriate name for what your body is doing and have learned how to control the nervous feeling by taking a breath—a breath that slows down the nervous autonomic response.

In this way, your emotions are tied to your thoughts, your body, and your behavior. Thoughts, body physiology, and behavior form the basis for how we function in the world, which shapes our world view. Emotions, then, are critical guides for the ways that we live our lives. They move us. Emotions give us direction and motivate our behavior, which determines how we interact with other people and situations, which forms the basis for our interpretation of life and its meaning.

The second part of the "movere" root of the word "emotions" is the idea that emotions are not meant to stick to us or stay inside of our bodies. Like clouds, they are supposed to move us in the moment, be experienced and dealt with as they move through us, and dissipate as they move along into the past.

However, everyone has been in a situation where the emotion they are experiencing cannot be dealt with right at that moment. You have to keep a straight face because it's not appropriate to laugh. You have to control yourself from throwing your arms around someone in gratitude because social norms prevent it. You can't yell at someone who has wronged you because of the possible consequences. When that happens, the emotion cloud sticks to you and hovers in the background of your day. It might pop up while you are trying to concentrate on writing an email or on the phone with a friend. The mind brings the memory of the context up into our consciousness over and over, causing us to experience the emotion over and over. We re-experience shame, amusement or disgust. We start to ruminate on it. The emotional cloud from the experience we had that morning overshadows the day, and we think about the context and feel the feeling when we are interacting with our coworkers, at the grocery store, picking up our children, and brushing our teeth before bed.

Some people use journaling to bring up the unprocessed emotions of the day and put them down on paper so that the feelings can be considered in a safe context. Once they are down on paper, we feel better. The cloud has been examined from all sides, pondered, felt fully, and now dissipates like it's supposed to. We stop thinking about it, and the emotion no longer tugs at the corners of the mind. Other people chat with friends or family members about experiences they had during the day. Others might work it out on the treadmill or in a boxing class. But the emotional clouds have to come out. They need to be tended to.

If we don't process our emotional clouds day-to-day, they thicken and become fog. The fog starts to hang over us. Now we are having new emotions today layered on top of all the rest of the emotions we had this week. By the time the work-week is over, we are exhausted by all the feelings and the thick fog we have built up. The longer this goes on—or the more intense the emotion is even if felt for a shorter time—the more the body-mind connection becomes oppressed.

To be sure, the body is still reacting to stimuli and contexts moment-to-moment, but its wisdom is listened to less and less. We just don't have the capacity to process it all and feel overwhelmed by all of the competing emotions vying for our attention. We might start to watch more TV or play video games in the evening. We stop talking with others about our day because it's just too much. We drink more alcohol or use more mind-altering substances—do more and more things to numb our feelings rather than feeling them. The variations in our heart beat ("heart rate variability") stop going up and down and stay at a chronically elevated state, correlated to many long-term health problems.

In TEAM, emotions come in through the Fire system. As I explained in the Fire Element question, the Pericardium is the protector of the Heart. So emotions first are experienced by the Pericardium and channeled to the Heart if circumstances allow them to be dealt with in that moment. If the Heart is busy attending to more pressing matters or if the Pericardium decides that circumstances do not allow for processing of the emotion at that moment, it stores the emotion in the courtyard of the solar plexus (there is that knot in your stomach again) for later when circumstances have changed. What happens next has some conflicting arguments in different TEAM texts, but I will try to explain it to the best of my ability and understanding.

If the emotion can't be dealt with after some time, the Pericardium solicits help from the Liver, who lives next door to the solar plexus under the right rib cage. In TEAM, it is the Liver's job to help regulate the smooth flow of Qi in the body. This includes emotional Qi. (The Pericardium and Liver are partnered as upper and lower body channels that are very closely linked for many reasons. This emotional processing business is one of them.) The Liver (under the right diaphragm) and Pericardium (on top of the left diaphragm) might elicit some deep breaths—pushing on the solar plexus—to try to clear the stuck emotion that way. We might also sigh, which is a deep breath and forced exhalation that strongly contracts the solar plexus and releases the shoulders.

If that is not effective, the Liver tries to regulate the emotion's passage to the associated superficial layers of the body tissues where it is almost, but not quite, out of the body. In the superficial layers (flesh, skin, bones, connective tissue, blood vessels), at least the emotion is not causing problems in the organs. But if that doesn't work or if the emotion keeps coming up and is not dealt with, the Liver and Pericardium might have to store the unexpressed emotion in its associated organ. Fear is housed long term in the Kidney/Urinary Bladder; worry in the Spleen/Stomach; grief in the Lung/Large Intestine; frustration/anger in the Liver/Gallbladder; and overjoy in the Heart/Small Intestine/Pericardium/San Jiao. (These are the correlations between emotions, organs, and tissue types that I discussed in the Five Element questions above.)

The longer we refuse to feel our feelings or push them down, commonly one (or both) of two things also happen. Either suppressed, frustrated, unexpressed, stagnant emotions start to come out as anger—we are yelling and screaming at everyone around us as the anger volcano erupts—and/or we feel so overwhelmed by the mountains of emotional clouds that it leads to hopelessness and depression. We feel completely stuck and don't know where to turn next. Moving out of the heavy fog feels pointless and overwhelming. I am sure that you already recognize that anger and hopelessness are emotions that dominate our society right now—the emotions of the Liver, yes, but also the result of all of the other emotions that we can't or don't experience and release.

In this way, long-term clouds of unexpressed worry, for example, are stored in the flesh and/or in the Spleen and Stomach. Those clouds might coalesce into heartburn or loud gurgling sounds when you eat or a constant knot in your upper stomach. (Conversely, when you journal, work with a talk therapist, exercise, meditate, or express your concerns to a friend, the worry is released from your Earth system. You crave less sugar. The heartburn feels better, the gurgles lessen, and the knot loosens.)

If we feel mostly anger, we walk around with tight shoulders and become increasingly inflexible as more and more emotional clouds fill up the space between our skin and our superficial tissues. If we feel mostly fear, we stop listening to signals around us (hearing worsens) because it is overwhelming to feel afraid all the time, and we might start to struggle with bladder control or kidney stones. If we seek joy and happiness all the time, we might become obsessed with feeling good and tip over into frenzied behaviors that are high-risk, high-reward in the moment but have negative long-term consequences such as overspending, unsafe sexual practices, or substances that make us feel really, really good for a short time.

It is important to note that happiness is a fleeting emotion and should be treated as such. The ideal emotional state is that of peace and satisfaction, according to the wisdom of TEAM. Being "centered" is not about being elated all the time. It is about recognizing that each emotion is a mini-experience that defines only that moment and should be held, felt, and released. The richness of our emotions give us the richness of the human experience and make life wondrous.

So the answer to your question is that emotions are important period—not just in TEAM but in life. Your emotions are valuable teachers that shape the way that you live your life. They color your world. They cloud or clarify your judgment and thinking. They distract or augment your experience as a human. And when they are not felt, emotions create pathology in your body. When they are experienced, considered and released, they create a healthy body and mind. In TEAM, there is a saying that unexpressed emotions are the root of all of the body's problems. Stagnant, raw, stuck emotions literally make you sick, and acupuncture can help you with that.

One of the most common comments that I hear from patients in response to acupuncture treatment is that they feel better. What I understand that to mean is not just that their pain is lessened, their ear ringing is quieter, or they feel less stuffy, but their feelings feel better. They feel lighter. They feel less burdened by their emotions and more able to take on life's challenges.

Acupuncture provides a pressure-release valve for the emotions you are having that don't otherwise have a place to bubble up and be released. If you are struggling to feel compassion for someone who has injured you, acupuncture can help to release that emotional hurt and give you a sense of distance so that forgiveness can start to be possible. If you are overwhelmed by sadness, it can release some of the grief. Acupuncture helps you to feel your feelings—defined by all the emotional names in your coloring box and changing from moment to moment just like the passing clouds—and find a place of peace in the midst of all of them.

### SEE ALSO

- "What is Five Element Theory?" *pg 23*
- "What does the Earth/Metal/Water/Wood/Fire Element (Phase) represent?" *pgs 23-46*
- "How does the thought theory of acupuncture differ from conventional medicine?" *pg 163*

## Q. How does an acupuncturist formulate a diagnosis and treatment plan?

This question could easily be placed organizationally in the "Logistics of Treatment" section, but I am putting it here because it seems to be one of the most confusing parts of seeing an acupuncturist. I think that is so because the foundations of TEAM are, quite literally, foreign to people who are not brought up in East Asian culture, and to some who are. While you have the ideas of Yin, Yang, Qi and Xue fresh in your mind, I think it makes sense to answer your questions about how TEAM theory is applied to the practical choices in clinic—what the acupuncturist does with the needles and related modalities and why. To do that, let's briefly touch on how we make a diagnosis and treatment plan in conventional medicine.

If I describe a set of symptoms like crushing chest pain that radiates down the left arm and into the jaw, shortness of breath, and a feeling of doom or fear, you might correctly tell me that you think the person experiencing those symptoms is having a heart attack. In medical education, we call that set of symptoms an "illness script." When we teach medical students to recognize a diagnosis like a heart attack, we use that set of symptoms together. We also use the stereotypical age (40's or 50's) and gender (male) to describe the person. It creates a stereotype in the medical student's mind of what someone looks like and what symptoms they will describe when they are experiencing that diagnosis. The medical student learns to listen to the patient (take a history) and to do a physical examination and put those components together to make a diagnosis (with or without testing).

As they become more and more skilled, they see people of different genders and ages having heart attacks, and they add those more unusual sets of symptoms to their mental file folder of what a heart attack looks like. For example, they might see a woman who is telling them not of crushing chest pain but of horrible nausea and upper abdominal pain: this person turns out to have a heart attack and they add that to their illness script file folder of what a heart attack looks like. In this way, they become more and more experienced about all the different variations on what a heart attack patient looks like and tells them about as their chief concern, and they learn to understand that a heart attack has a "classic presentation" but can show up in a wide variety of ways.

The diagnosis is the basis for the treatment plan. In our heart attack patient above, they would need to take medication immediately to help prevent blood clots from forming in the area where the plaque has likely pulled away from the blood vessel wall, causing the heart attack. The person also needs to see a cardiologist immediately and go to a cath lab so that the blockage can be unblocked. The medical student learns why a heart attack happens specifically in the body, the pharmacology that needs to be given to prevent the situation from getting worse, and the physical anatomical intervention that needs to be done to stabilize the patient.

Similarly in TEAM, the acupuncturist will listen to you and take your history. However, the way that the body is put together in TEAM is a little different from conventional medicine. The illness scripts are not the same.

If I told my medical students that a person has thirst but no desire to drink, a hard time getting out of bed in the morning, a foggy head and heavy limbs, and no appetite until 11:00 AM, they would not put that information together as an illness script and make a diagnosis. That set of symptoms doesn't amount to anything in conventional medicine. However, all of my acupuncture students would tell me that person has Spleen Qi Deficiency with Dampness, which is an illness script diagnosis in TEAM. They would confirm that diagnosis by feeling a slippery pulse in the Spleen position and seeing that the person's tongue was puffy with prominent teeth marks/scalloping on both sides of the tongue.

The treatment of Spleen Qi Deficiency with Dampness is to 1. strengthen the Spleen Qi, and 2. dry Dampness. This is done with diet, acupuncture, and herbal medicines. But the source or root cause of the diagnosis is generally overthinking or worry. I see it a lot, ironically, in the students themselves because ruminating on your thoughts (like studying or working on a big project) is very similar to ruminating on your food in TEAM. That rumination causes the Qi to get stuck. In German, the word for this concept translates as "thought carousel" (Gedankenkarussell), which I think is an apt description of how your mind goes round and round, but you can't get off the carousel and make a decision about what to do next.

Practitioners who do acupuncture—especially those practitioners who are trained in the technique but have limited training in the theory of TEAM—get into trouble, in my opinion, when they try to use acupuncture to treat patients in the context of conventional medicine instead of the context of TEAM. It just doesn't work as well or as consistently as using the acupuncture technique within the context of TEAM. I tend to see a lot of patients in my practice who have been to clinicians who are minimally trained in the technique of placing acupuncture needles in the skin (like dry needling or trigger point therapy) but who are frustrated because they are not getting good results. The relief of pain lasts, for example, for a few days but doesn't really go away. While I don't have scientific data to back up this statement, I suspect it is because the practitioner is trying to help the patient with acupuncture or related techniques but is doing it in the context of their original training (medical, chiropractic, physical therapy, etc.) rather than in the context of TEAM.

I have had to think for a long time to come up with a good metaphor for you, but I think this might help. Two people are trying to figure out how to get out of an escape room. The instructions in the escape room are in French and require French spelling of words to get to the next clues. One of the people in the escape room speaks American sign language (ASL), and the other speaks Korean. There is no translator. Neither person can follow the puzzle and come up with the appropriate French answer because their context is ASL and Korean. They might be able to make a little progress, but coming up with the clue-specific word in French will be impossible because they don't speak the French language. Similarly, I don't think a clinician can use acupoints to their fullest potential without understanding the context of TEAM.

Finally, it is important to know that TEAM is whole-person medicine, and this is critical for both diagnosis and treatment decisions. The diagnosis or diagnoses will reflect where the imbalances are in your body, mind and emotions.

In conventional medicine, you might have diagnoses of migraine headaches, tight neck and shoulders, menstrual irregularities, and abdominal pain. You will get different specific diagnoses for each of them and then a separate treatment for each one of them. Rather than treating each of them separately, an acupuncturist will look at all of those conventional medicine diagnoses as symptoms of a root cause and then treat that root cause collectively—in this case, Wood over-controlling Earth.

This is, in my opinion, the most important difference between conventional medicine and TEAM. Conventional medicine is focused on finding your diagnosis by reducing the other possibilities until you are left with one right answer—one right illness script that is confirmed by physical exam findings and lab or radiographic findings—for each problem that you have. It then repeats this same exercise with another set of illness scripts and findings to come up with a diagnosis for every other problem that you have.

The organization of conventional medicine is structured around this thought process and is the reason we have experts in joints, in nerves, in emotional health, in digestive functions, in hearts, etc. Each expert performs a deep dive into their organ system and knows the relevant illness scripts in great detail. The primary care providers are the guides in this system and have to know a LOT of things about a LOT of things in order to help you get to the person who can figure out the unusual issues you are having.

TEAM looks at all of your concerns and problems as a part of one big pot of stew. It considers the components of the problem stew (vegetables over here, broth over here, meat over here) to get a sense of how the components are affecting each other, but then it unites the separate problems under one primary diagnosis, viewing the components as parts of a cohesive whole. It treats the problem stew by adding herbal seasonings, Yin water, and Yang heat to make the stew work together more cohesively, in exactly the right proportions that you need to become balanced again. It stirs the stew together with Qi, which moves the component parts together so that each bite is balanced and pleasant.

The acupuncture points we use and herbal medicines we prescribe are intended to treat you—all of you and all of your concerns—at the same time. This is why, when patients ask me why I am using a specific acupuncture point ("What's that point for?"), I tell them, "It's for you." I then explain how all of the points are working together and that each point is part of the function of the collective rather than a single point working in isolation from the other points. Like the players in a team sport, the points are assigned to different positions, but they have to work together in order to accomplish the end result successfully. Herbal formulas are similarly prescribed for the root cause of your issues rather than one herb for each problem. The herbal formula and acupoint selection are conceived as a collective treatment, tailored to your specific needs, based on your individual, whole-person diagnosis.

## SEE ALSO

- "What is Five Element Theory?" *pg 23*
- "Why does the acupuncturist want to see my tongue and feel my wrists?" *pg 130*
- "How does the thought theory of acupuncture differ from conventional medicine?" *pg 163*

.

# CHAPTER TWO

# HOW DOES ACUPUNCTURE WORK?

## Q. What is acupuncture?

Acupuncture as a technique can be very generally defined as a treatment modality that uses thin sterile needles (about the diameter of the hair on your head) placed into the skin, connective tissues, or muscles to treat a wide variety of medical, psychological, and emotional concerns. The needles are generally left in place for a period of 15-45 minutes, after which they are removed and the recipient goes on their way. That said, there are variations on almost everything that I just asserted in the definition above.

The needles might be used to brush or scrape the skin instead of being inserted into the skin. The needles might be inserted and then immediately removed. They might be inserted and retained for several days, such as in battlefield acupuncture, or weeks, such as in auricular acupuncture. The needles might be replaced with a tool called a "teshin" which does not penetrate the skin but instead creates very specific pressure on an acupoint—a wonderful and useful technique for children or people with a very low pain threshold. (More on acupoints soon.)

Gentle electrical current may be passed between two or more needles in a technique called "electrical stimulation" or "e-stim." The needles might be inserted into a spastic muscle to elicit a twitch response, causing the muscle to relax, or into specific pressure points as in "dry needling." The needles might be thicker or thinner in diameter, longer or shorter in length, or free form or attached to adhesive.

The placement of the acupuncture needles offers yet another level of variety and options. Needles may be placed in areas all over the body using meridian maps. They might be placed in points that are anatomically defined but off the meridian lines ("extra points") or in palpable, tender spots on the skin that tend to move around ("Ah shi" points).

Acupuncture also conceives of microsystems. These microsystems on the scalp, ear, abdomen, face, hand and other areas can be used to treat the whole body using reflection sites. Extremely small superficial needles may be placed and retained, most commonly in or on the ear microsystem. These needles are generally less than 1 mm in diameter and 1-3 mm long and are applied using a small plastic attachment to the dull end of the needle surrounded by an adhesive substance like a sticky note. These retained needles are intended to prolong the effects of treatment as the person stimulates them over the next few days or weeks.

In the United States, Great Britain, and Australia, "acupuncture" colloquially refers to the TEAM profession as a whole and includes several other modalities that do not involve acupuncture needles. In the United States, these include gua sha, tui na, moxibustion, diet, herbal medicine, movement and exercise, and mindfulness practices. Being a licensed acupuncturist means that a person has at least some training in all of these modalities.

**SEE ALSO**

- "What are acupuncture channels or meridians? What are acupoints?" *pg 65*

- "What is Traditional East Asian Medicine (TEAM)?" *pg 13*

- "What is the history of acupuncture in the West?" *pg 159*

- "Where do the needles go?" *pg 133*

- "What other kinds of things can an acupuncturist do?" *pg 145*

## Q. What are acupuncture channels or meridians? What are acupoints?

There are 12 primary organs in TEAM that govern the body's functions. They are arranged in Yin-Yang pairs (also called "Zang-Fu"). Not coincidentally, there are 12 main meridians or channels that connect those organs to other parts of the body, to tissue types, and to sensory organs. You have one of these channels on the left side of your body and another one on the right side of your body. For example, you have a Heart channel on your left arm and your right arm and a Stomach channel on your left leg and your right leg.

There are 2 additional channels with multiple points along them that are not linked to a specific organ. They are the Ren Mai (Conception vessel) that runs along the center midline of the body and the Du Mai (Governing vessel) that runs along the back midline of the body. Because these channels are right in the middle of your body, there is only one of each of them.

The meridians function as an organizing highway map along which 361 of the acupuncture points ("acupoints") can be found.

The channel pathways and acupoint locations are defined anatomically (in the groove between a particular bone and a muscle, for example). In this way, the acupuncturist can find the channel and acupuncture points along the channel by palpating the anatomy of the patient.

## SEE ALSO

- "What is Five Element Theory?" *pg 23*
- "What does the Earth/Metal/Water/Wood/Fire Element (Phase) represent?" *pgs 23-46*
- "Where do the needles go?" *pg 133*
- "What other kinds of things can an acupuncturist do?" *pg 145*

## Q. How many acupuncture points are there?

The short answer is that there are thousands of acupuncture points on your body. Virtually any spot can be used at one time or another as an acupuncture point. Acupuncture points are arranged into two big categories: those that are on channels and those that are not.

## Points on Meridians

On the 14 channels or meridians, there are 361 discrete acupoints. They have names in East Asian languages like "Rushing Qi" or "Sea of Blood," but in the West, we name the points according to the meridian and the numbered sequence along the meridian. Instead of "Rushing Qi," we call it Stomach 30 and abbreviate it with a 2-letter designation, ST30. This is kind of like "Interstate 90, Exit 47." It tells you which road you are on (the "Stomach" road) and also how far along the road you need to travel in order to get there (the 30th point on the meridian).

## Points not on Meridians

### Extra points

There are many more points that are not on channels. Some of these are called "extra points" and are named by their Chinese name. For example, there is a point under the earlobe called "An Mian" and is commonly used for sleep. It is easy to remember because it sounds like "Ambien," which is a common sleep medication. These extra points are all over the body and have a wide variety of functions.

### Microsystems points

Then there are non-channel microsystem points on the ear, points on the hands, points on the feet, points on the abdomen, and points on the head. Using these microsystems, you can impact the entire body. There are points, for example, on your hand that can impact everything from your head to your belly to your ankles. These points number in the hundreds.

You can think of microsystems like a handheld street map. The city of London that you see on the map is much smaller than the actual city itself, yet there is a representation of streets, waterways and buildings that can be used as a guide to the actual city. Similarly, the map of your entire body can be found in small representations on your ear or your hand. That small map can be used to access the larger organs and meridians on the larger body. This is particularly helpful in situations where a person has pain in multiple places on their shoulder. Rather than using body points on the front, back and sides of their actual shoulder, you can efficiently treat the entire shoulder using the "shoulder point" on their ear, hand, foot, scalp, or abdomen.

*Ah shi points*

Finally there are non-channel points called "Ah shi" points. When you say the word "Ah shi" out loud, it sounds like "ouchy," which is what these points are used for. If you feel around on your forearm or your leg, you will find some spots that are surprisingly painful—more so than the other skin around them. In acupuncture, that spot is an indication that there is something out of balance related to that point that your body is asking for help resolving. An acupuncturist might put a needle in that spot or into a spot on another part of your body to help that imbalance resolve.

I like to think of Ah shi points as smoke signals showing me where there are small, smoldering fires. They need to be addressed before they grow into a big fire. Since everybody's body is a little different, the places that the smoke signals go up will be unique and might change over time as the body changes, ages, responds to various stressors, and gets sicker or more healthy.

**SEE ALSO**

- "What are acupuncture channels or meridians? What are acupoints?" *pg 65*
- "Where do the needles go?" *pg 133*

## Q. How does the acupuncturist pick which acupoints to use?

Depending on a person's health concerns and the organ systems or meridians involved in those concerns, an acupuncturist will select the acupoints needed to rebalance the system. This is a vague answer and likely unsatisfying. I will use some examples so that I can be more specific. However, the subtle logic of needle prescription is something that I continue to learn year after year after year of practice. It is the art of being an acupuncturist and not easily explained.

If you have hives on your skin and are sneezing from allergies, your acupuncturist might treat the Lung and Large Intestine channels—the Metal channels. Remember that Metal is used to treat skin and immune system problems. If the acupuncturist is using Five Element Theory, they might use Water points on the Fire channel to cool the Fire that is making the hives itchy and red and irritating your nose. They might use Metal points to support the Water. They might use acupoint LI4 because it is the command point of the head and face and is also a Metal point.

If you have issues with a sprained ankle, a Five Element acupuncturist might use the Liver or Gallbladder channels (Wood is associated with tendons and connective tissue) and your Kidney or Urinary Bladder channels (Water is associated with your bones). They might use the Water points on the Wood channels and the

Wood points on the Water channels. Not surprisingly, the command point for the tendons is on the Gall Bladder meridian and would probably be used in this case. The acupuncturist might also use acupoints to move stagnant Qi and Blood, which contribute to the pain of a sprained ankle.

In other theoretical constructs, the meridians can be thought to connect to each other in sets of four. In each of the sets of four, there are two channels that are on the upper body (arm) and two channels on the lower body (leg). They are paired by the Yin arm channel and Yin leg channel to make the Yin half of the set. The Yang arm channel and Yang leg channel make the Yang half of the set.

The LU, LI, SP and ST make a set called Tai Yin (LU + SP) and Yang Ming (LI + ST).

The HT, SI, KI, and UB channels make up the Shao Yin (HT + KI) and Tai Yang (SI + UB) set.

The PC, SJ, LV, and GB meridians are the Jue Yin (PC + LV) and Shao Yang (SJ + GB) quartet.

Using our example of hives and allergies above, the acupuncturist would likely add acupoints from the Spleen and Stomach channels on your legs to balance the arm acupoints they are using on your Lung and Large Intestine channels.

Again, please don't get too stressed about the details of how things are put together, but I do want to give you a sense that your acupuncturist is thinking very conscientiously about where exactly they are placing needles for you and how they are rebalancing your system with all of these relationships. It's complicated!

| YIN ORGAN & CHANNEL | YANG ORGAN & CHANNEL | ARM OR LEG? | TISSUE TYPES | SENSORY ORGANS |
|---|---|---|---|---|
| Lung (LU) | Large Intestine (LI) | Arm | Skin | Nose |
| Spleen (SP) | Stomach (ST) | Leg | Flesh, muscle | Mouth |
| Heart (HT) | Small Intestine (SI) | Arm | Blood & blood vessels | Tongue |
| Kidney (KI) | Urinary Bladder (UB or BL) | Leg | Bones | Ears |
| Pericardium (PC) | Triple Heater (TH) or San Jiao (SJ) | Arm | Blood & blood vessels | Tongue |
| Liver (LV or LR) | Gallbladder (GB) | Leg | Tendons | Eyes |

## SEE ALSO

- "What are acupuncture channels or meridians? What are acupoints?" *pg 65*
- "How many acupuncture points are there?" *pg 66*
- "Where do the needles go?" *pg 133*
- "What other kinds of practitioners can use acupuncture needles?" *pg 149*
- "What is the difference between acupuncture and dry needling?" *pg 151*

## Q. What does acupuncture actually do?

### Self-healing mechanisms

First, acupuncture activates your body's self healing mechanisms. This might sound like mumbo-jumbo, but your body is actually very wise. When you cut your finger, your body does not need instructions about how to put your finger back together. Regardless of how deep the cut (assuming you didn't cut your finger off), how many tissue layers, whether or not blood vessels are involved, and whether the skin is thick or thin in that area, your body knows how to fix all of the layers and keep your finger functioning.

Some of this includes automatic mechanisms that go into play when the inside of a blood vessel is disrupted, which activates the clotting system, tells white blood cells to come into the area, and starts to make your blood vessels leaky so your tissues swell and start to fill up the cut or hole created. Your body also sends a nerve signal from the cut to your brain, letting your brain know you've been injured. Acupuncture has been shown to boost your body's ability to fix itself at many of the autonomic steps I just described.

### Endogenous opioid system

What happens when you can't stop to take care of that cut? What if you cut your finger while trying to run away from a bear, or you twist your ankle in the middle of a busy intersection but you need to get out of the way of oncoming traffic? Your body doesn't stop running just because you cut your finger. Your brain takes in that information but it deprioritizes it in favor of getting away from the bear or out of traffic. It does this through a system of chemical communications collectively known as the endogenous opioid system. Yup, that's the same messenger system that opioid medications were designed to treat.

As it turns out, the second thing that acupuncture does is affect your endogenous opioid system. It is through this system that acupuncture has such potent effects on pain, but without all the nasty (and sometimes fatal!) side effects of opioid medications like hydrocodone or fentanyl.

This might be well and good when you think about a twisted ankle or cut on your finger—pretty simple really—but how does acupuncture help with diabetes, heart problems, anxiety and depression, or other long-term issues?

## *Gene expression and translation*

In the medical literature, acupuncture has also been shown to change the way genes are expressed and translated into proteins and other signals, reduce inflammation, increase blood flow, and alter the biochemical environment of tissues around an acupuncture needle.

In addition, acupuncture has been shown to change the concentration of different peripheral chemical messengers that conduct signals between nerves and other tissues and to change the ability of nerve cells to carry information from the body tissues to the brain and the spinal cord. In other words, it can influence the way your brain receives information from the body and the way that your brain sends information to the body.

Acupuncture also influences emotional processing areas of the brain like the amygdala and can reverse some of the nerve signaling issues in chronic dementia.

Cell studies have even shown that cells rearrange their internal architecture (cytoskeleton) in response to acupuncture needles. In other words, cells move their cell "bones" around to orient them differently when an acupuncture needle is present and stimulating them.

We are only beginning to understand the depths of what acupuncture can do at a cellular level in the conventional medical literature, but even with that, acupuncture has a broad range of very real physiological effects on the body.

**SEE ALSO**

- "Does acupuncture treat pain?" *pg 93*
- "What can acupuncture not do?" *pg 74*

## Q. What can acupuncture not do?

Acupuncture should not be your first choice in emergency situations. For life-threatening situations, go to an emergency room, not an acupuncturist's office. If your appendix is ruptured, go to the emergency room. If you cannot breathe, go to the emergency room. If you are in a car accident and you have neck and back pain, go to the emergency room—and then think about acupuncture after you make sure nothing is broken or ripped.

If you're having excruciating pain in your head that came on suddenly or a change in your ability to talk, see, or move your limbs, then that is a trip to the emergency room. If you have chest pain that feels like an elephant is sitting on your chest with numbness/pain in your left arm, please for the love of all that is good and holy, go to the emergency room. Acupuncture is not capable of setting a broken bone but will help it to heal. First, you need a trip to the emergency room to get it set and cast or splinted.

Those are emergencies. Conventional medicine is truly great for emergencies. If there is ever a question of whether or not something is an emergency, a trip to the emergency room—or at the very least a call to your primary care provider—is always the best choice.

Similarly, do not count on acupuncture to save your life if you have other serious non-emergency room conditions like cancer or heart, kidney or liver failure. It is a good adjunct to conventional treatment for reasons we have already discussed, but at this time, I would not recommend acupuncture as the only treatment for the cancer or organ failure itself.

Similarly, acupuncture is not a quick fix for medical conditions that have developed slowly over long periods of time like dementia, advanced diabetes-related problems (nerve damage, kidney failure, etc.), "bone on bone" pain in the joints or spine, or serious lung or kidney problems. Some of the symptoms of these long-term, chronic issues can be helped with acupuncture, but acupuncture treatment should be done in conjunction with conventional medical therapy. Likewise, Crohn's disease and ulcerative colitis symptoms can be supported with acupuncture, but you should not ignore conventional medical therapies for these and similar issues.

I am including this last part a bit tongue-in-cheek, but you'd be surprised what people come to me expecting acupuncture to do for them. So to be clear...

Acupuncture cannot change your height, your personality, your upbringing, your boss, or your spouse.

The 60 minutes you spend getting an acupuncture treatment each week cannot overcome the unhealthy choices you make for the other 167 hours of that week like eating fast food, drinking too much caffeine or alcohol, not exercising, and not sleeping.

Sadly, getting acupuncture does not mean you can eat all the ice cream you want and still maintain a healthy body and blood sugar levels. (The acupuncture researchers should really get on this!)

It cannot make your hair regrow overnight or make all your wrinkles disappear in one session—although it can help both of those things over time.

It is not an excuse to not take care of yourself or to ignore the solid advice of a medical provider working in conventional medicine which, like acupuncture, is based on the scientific observation of what happens when you do or do not follow that advice. It's pretty amazing, but it is unfortunately not a magical panacea.

---

**SEE ALSO**

- "What does acupuncture actually do?" *pg 72*

---

## Q. Does acupuncture heal?

The way that our brain communicates with the rest of our tissues is by electricity. The electrical signals are transformed into chemical signals, which then elicit some kind of chemical reaction at the end point of communication. These reactions might stimulate a gate to open in a cell membrane, create a chemical reaction that causes muscles to contract or to relax, or change gene expression within the cell.

Similarly, the flow of electrical and chemical signals in and out of cells impacts the behavior of cells and tissues around them. Your body's abilities to make blood clots in response to a cut on your finger, to secrete digestive enzymes into your stomach and small intestine in response to the food you are eating, and to focus your eyes on something close to you and then farther away are all determined by electrical and chemical messengers.

When you insert a needle from the air into someone's body, there is a small electrical gradient that is set up simply because of the difference in temperature: electrons will move along a metal needle just because the outside air is 75 degrees and your body temperature is 98 degrees. Those signals are even stronger when we hook up acupuncture needles to a gentle a form of energy that comes from the presence of or the movement of charged particles like electrons and protons (electroacupuncture). Similarly, the small injury from the introduction of the needle causes a cascade of chemical messengers in the tissues around the needle.

That acupuncture needle tip starts to change the electrical signaling in that particular area of the body, which is translated from one area of the body to the next because we are made of water with salts in it. Salt water conducts electricity. This means that the small electrical signal changes I have created by putting a needle in your wrist will travel gently up your arm to your elbow, to your shoulder, and to your neck, etc. Because all the chemical and electrical signals going on in that area can be influenced by the acupuncture needle, the entire milieu of that area can be changed by the insertion of an acupuncture needle.

While it is difficult to define "healing," acupuncture influences the biochemistry of the body locally around the needle and farther away, similarly to the way the brain influences the nerves that come out of it and influences the movement of your toes. When the biochemistry changes, cells behave differently, pathways are activated or turned off, chemical signals enact a series of changes, etc., all of which add up to "healing."

So I would say that acupuncture assists the body in doing what it knows how to do. It is a helpful nudge in the direction of improving functioning of a tissue type or organ system. But I would not say that acupuncture alone, without the help of the body's intrinsic wisdom, heals all by itself.

### SEE ALSO

- "What does acupuncture actually do?" *pg 72*
- "Will acupuncture help my problem?" *pg 87*

## Q. Is acupuncture pseudoscience or real?

Acupuncture is absolutely real. There are hundreds of thousands of articles on acupuncture, how it works, and what it does in peer-reviewed scientific journals in different languages and countries all over the world.

I think one of the reasons this question persists is that acupuncture is taught in the context of a medical paradigm that is very different from conventional medicine. Words like "Liver Qi stagnation" are not heard in a regular doctor's office and can be off-putting because we typically think of medicine as a science. "Qi" is not a science word.

It was this issue that made it so hard for me to learn about acupuncture as a conventional medical doctor. After all my years of conventional medical training (2 years Master's in Physiology and Biophysics + 4 years of medical school + 4 years of general surgery residency), I thought that I had a pretty good understanding of anatomy and how the body was put together and how the parts work individually and as a whole.

When I started studying acupuncture, I found it easy to memorize the acupoint locations and functions and how they fit into the East Asian medicine theory. I had felt the effects of acupuncture on the pain in my body, but I didn't really think the channels were real in the same way that connecting structures like lymph and blood vessels were real.

I thought about the meridians as a convenient map that linked acupoints with similar functions together in a way that made it easier for clinicians to conceptualize and treat people. Yes, there was a link between them in terms of function, but I had never seen a meridian in the cadaver lab or in any patient I had cut open on the operating table or stitched back together in the trauma bay.

I then was in a weekend seminar with a Japanese teacher who had been practicing acupuncture for 50 years. He had me on a table in a room in front of ~200 people and was lecturing to them. He felt my pulses while still talking to the learners and then put one needle in my leg in the Gallbladder channel. I felt as if a warm magic marker were drawing a line up my leg following that channel. As you can see, that is a zig-zag of a pathway—no nerve or blood vessel does that.

At the moment when the warm magic marker reached the end of the channel by my eye, he looked down and smiled at me. He was still holding the handle of the needle which was inserted in my leg with his fingertips. That warm sensation was the Qi of the channel opening up and flowing. He was feeling it move as guided by the acupuncture needle and knew when it had reached the end of the channel.

Gallbladder Meridian

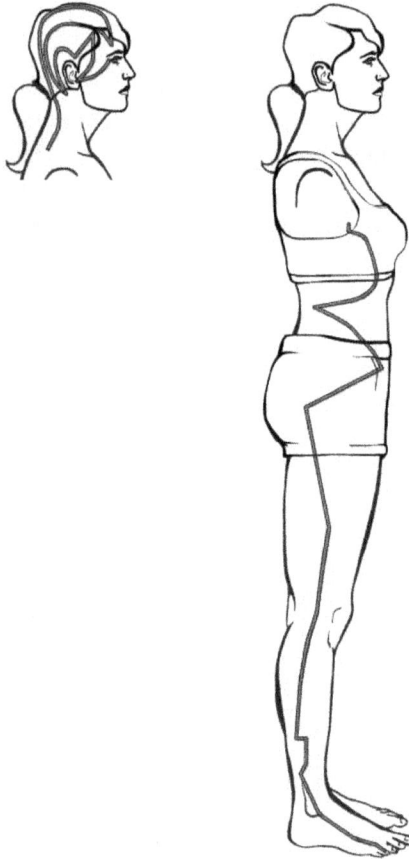

In that moment, I realized the channels were and are just as real as any nerve, muscle, or blood vessel that I have dissected, cut, or

sewn. Even though I have talked about that moment many times to colleagues or patients or medical students or attendees listening to me lecture, the revelation of the realness of acupuncture in that moment still elicits a strong response in my body—makes me choke up a bit and brings tears to my eyes.

Just like it took the invention of the microscope to identify bacteria and the invention of an ultrasound to see blood flowing through the heart and blood vessels, I think we haven't invented the technology to be able to "see" Qi yet. We are getting closer, but we just don't have the right instruments yet. But yes, from my experience as a patient and as a practitioner, acupuncture points and acupuncture meridians are very real.[1]

## SEE ALSO

- "How does an acupuncturist formulate a diagnosis and treatment plan?" *pg 56*
- "What does acupuncture actually do?" *pg 72*
- "Is acupuncture just placebo?" *pg 82*
- "How does the thought theory of acupuncture differ from conventional medicine?" *pg 163*

---

1   There is some interesting work being done by Poney Chiang and colleagues that is beginning to explain why we don't see Qi channels in cadavers and many other people are looking at the anatomical relationship between nerves, blood vessels and acupoints. See the References section for more details.

## Q. Is acupuncture just placebo?

I love this question. Let's tackle the issue of defining placebo first.

### *What is placebo?*

In conventional medicine and science, placebo has come to mean "it's all in your mind." It's the idea that when you think something will help, it has an impact on whether or not it actually does help.

When you are doing an experiment and want to isolate whether or not, for example, a particular pill is helping someone's blood pressure to come down, you want to try to eliminate all the things that might confuse your results. You want to know about the effects of the pill only. So scientists have developed methods that try to eliminate anything that might "confound" the results. They randomize the people getting the pill and those that don't, they try to make the pretend ("placebo") pill and the real ("verum") pill groups as similar to each other as possible, and they try not to give any clues whether a person is getting the real or the pretend drug. They definitely don't say things like "I think this will really help you."

These placebo-controlled experiments work really well when you are talking about pharmaceutical medications. (Drugs only have to work a very small percentage points better than placebo—sometimes only single digits better.) Placebo control doesn't work so well when you want to check whether or not physical therapy will help shoulder pain or whether yoga therapy helps with balance. You can't really give someone fake physical therapy or fake yoga.

The scientific community acknowledges, by trying to control its effects, that placebo is very powerful. In fact, there are many studies that show how powerful placebo is—how powerful the mind is in healing the body.

### *The mind is a powerful healing tool.*

One study that I find particularly intriguing involves people who needed knee surgery for osteoarthritis, which is inflammation in the knee from wear and tear. The surgeons did actual knee surgery for osteoarthritis (either debridement of the joint or lavage) in some of the patients in the study. For other patients, the surgeons just made the incisions in the skin and then sewed the cuts on the skin back up. They did not do any of the actual surgical work on the knee. It was a placebo surgery for these patients. The researchers then followed all the patients for two years to see if there were any differences between people who had real versus placebo surgery.

There was no difference in outcomes or knee pain or knee function between the 165 people in the different groups. In other words, at no point in the two years did the people who had actual surgery report less pain or better function than the placebo group!

So what happened to make the people who didn't have "real" surgery better? How did small cuts on their skin and no surgery on their knees result in less pain and better function?

Even more interesting is the question of is "real" knee surgery really necessary or is the process of thinking you are going to be helped (placebo) all that is needed? Is real surgery even doing anything or is it just the patient's mind that does the healing—just thinking that you will be better from a surgery might be what is making it so.

As a doctor, this is really, really shocking to wrap my head around. I don't think it is a simple yes or no answer. I can't imagine that not taking a brain tumor out of a person's head or sewing up a hole in someone's colon is not helpful and needed. The surgeon in these situations is doing something that is absolutely necessary. But based on the research I mentioned above, I also have to acknowledge that a substantial part of the healing process (after the brain tumor is out or the colon perforation is closed up) is the person's thoughts and feelings around the surgery and their belief that they will be better after the procedure. The mind is part of healing.

Understanding the role that placebo has in conventional medical therapies like medication and surgery, now let's consider the question of whether placebo is also important in the context of acupuncture.

## Placebo in acupuncture

Scientists have designed studies of pretend ("sham") acupuncture, real ("verum") acupuncture, and no acupuncture. Most of the sham acupuncture involves holding a little device over the acupuncture point and putting pressure on the acupoint instead of inserting a needle into the point. These devices are essentially acupressure.

In studies like this, there is commonly either a small difference or no difference between sham and verum acupuncture. In studies that use different kinds of sham acupuncture, the differences tend to be a bit bigger. When the studies are done on larger populations of people, the differences become more pronounced. This has to do with sample size statistics and is proof that there is a difference. It just takes larger numbers of people in the study to show it definitively.

Because some people have a hard time "believing" in acupuncture (believing implies it is a religion or leap of faith instead of having scientific basis so I am not a fan of that term), they have a hard time conceptualizing that acupuncture would be anything more than tricks the mind is playing on the body. As we have discussed in other questions, that is just not true. There are just too many scientific studies that show acupuncture is "doing stuff" in the body.

## What does this mean for you?

As a person who is thinking about getting acupuncture, you are likely thinking about it because you have an issue that you would like to have resolved. You have pain or anxiety or digestive issues or problems sleeping. You want a solution to your problem, and you are curious about the answer to this question because you want to know if acupuncture can help you.

So let's pretend that acupuncture has not been around for thousands of years and used to treat millions of people for many, many different medical problems for a moment. Let's also pretend that acupuncture is engaging the placebo effect only.

Would you not want to engage every part of you to help you get better? Do you not want your mind to help your body resolve this health concern that you have? Do you not want your brain to assist in your recovery and healing?

So if I have a medical treatment option that has an extremely low risk of any significant side effects, is relaxing, is almost always painless (or minimally painful for a few seconds), has many proven health benefits, and engages your mind in your healing and ongoing health, would it not make sense to use it?

For myself, I want to use everything available to me to keep my body strong, fit and healthy: my diet, my sleep, my lifestyle, my exercise, and my mind (my placebo effect). I "set my mind" to it and use my mind to help me in every area of my life, including my health.

So the answer to this question is that yes, acupuncture is more than placebo. And also that placebo is a part of the healing process regardless of what kind of medicine you decide to use for your health issues and concerns.

## SEE ALSO

- "What is acupuncture?" *pg 63*
- "Is acupuncture pseudoscience or real?" *pg 78*
- "References" *pg 181*

# CHAPTER THREE

# HOW CAN ACUPUNCTURE HELP ME?

## Q. Will acupuncture help my problem?

This is an interesting question because acupuncture helps...not all the things, but almost all of the things that humans experience in their physical, mental and emotional bodies.

Feeling overworked, stressed, overwhelmed, tired, and wired? Acupuncture can help that.

Feeling pain in your joints, your belly, your head, your heart, or anywhere else in or on your body, even when they can't find anything on X Rays or scans or scopes or bloodwork? Acupuncture can help with that.

Can't sleep, feel exhausted when you wake up, or have an afternoon slump? Napping necessary to get through the day? Wake up multiple times in the night and your mind starts racing? Snoring waking you up or waking your sleeping partner? Acupuncture can help with all of that.

Digestive problems? Can't go or go too much or too often or too loud or too painful or too much or too little? Loud gurgling sounds in your belly? Passing gas or burping? Heartburn, nausea, indigestion, upset stomach? Acupuncture can really help with that.

Anxious and on high alert all the time? Can't focus or pay attention? Find yourself asking the same questions over and over and not retaining the answers? Feeling hopeless, lost, directionless, stuck, or depressed? Acupuncture can help with that.

Have a cold or flu? Coughing, sneezing, and stuffy head? Sore throat and not sure if it is allergies or you'll need to call in sick tomorrow? Call an acupuncturist immediately. Every time I've done that—even knowing how amazing acupuncture is because I practice this medicine—I'm blown away by how quickly I get over my symptoms and how much more easily my body recovers. So yeah, acupuncture can help with all of that.

My personal experience with acupuncture is that it makes me feel more like my best self: the calm, confident, grounded, capable me that I know I am at my core but sometimes struggle to find when I am in pain, exhausted, overwhelmed, or distracted by life stuff. So while it will help my ankle pain, the numbness in my arm when it flares up, or a stomach flu or a summer cold, the real benefit of acupuncture to me is that it helps me live optimally in my best mind, my best emotions, and my best body.

## Q. Can you use acupuncture as preventative medicine?

In previous times, an acupuncturist was paid not when the patient was ill but when they were well. Thus the financial impetus was to keep the person healthy. It was considered the job of the acupuncturist to prevent problems. If the acupuncturist did not correctly see an event on the horizon and prevent it from happening, they were morally and fiscally responsible for rectifying the situation.

(How radically would healthcare change if we did the same in conventional medicine?!) In that context, it is easy to see the benefits of using acupuncture for prevention of problems.

## Physical health benefits

If your toe didn't hurt, you would not change your gait. If you didn't change your gait, your knee and hip would not be asked to bear the brunt of your walking. If you didn't develop pain when walking, you might be more mobile overall and more keen to exercise. If you were more interested in exercise, you might be more aware of your eating patterns and less likely to develop sugar addictions. The sugar addiction leads to chronic elevated blood sugar levels which leads to diabetes which leads, in combination with the sedentary lifestyle that includes more bacon and less salads, to heart disease which leads to a heart attack which leads to an even more sedentary lifestyle which makes you more likely to develop... You see where I'm going here. Preventing issues from arising is key. It is the key to maintaining one's health and thereby one's longevity—one's pleasure in living a long, fulfilling life. And get that toe evaluated!

## Mental and emotional health benefits

I think it is important to reinforce here that mental health and emotional health are critical facets of whole-person health. My experience as a patient of acupuncture and a practitioner of acupuncture is that what is happening in the mind absolutely cannot be distanced from what is happening in the body. This is the profoundest and most amazing part (in my opinion) of acupuncture. Thoughts shape reality. What I mean is this—

If our thoughts are continuously drawn to grief and sorrow, we get stuck in that pattern and begin to see the world as a sorrowful place, expecting loss and separation. If we are drawn to fear, we see the world as a fearful place and wait for harm to come our way. If we see things through a lens of sunshine and roses, we view the world as an idyllic landscape and are surprised when others don't behave in a fairyland manner. As I have mentioned before, it is the range of human emotion that gives life meaning, and our emotions have a direct impact on our health. Acupuncture helps us to process our emotions—to experience them and then let them go. The emotions don't become stuck and therefore don't become a pattern. We are able to clearly see events in our lives from a place of balance rather than through a limited, single-emotion lens.

The benefits, then, of regular acupuncture are preventing problems from arising and preserving one's health: mentally, emotionally, and physically.

### *What should I ask for?*

If you are going to see an acupuncturist for prevention of problems, the practitioner will want to hear about how you are functioning currently and what health issues you may have encountered previously in your life. They will ask about your diet, lifestyle, stressors, sleep, and activity. All of this will give them clues about where you might be more or less likely to develop health problems in the future and what steps might be needed to prevent them from happening.

## SEE ALSO

- "Why are emotions so important in Traditional East Asian Medicine?" *pg 46*

- "What does acupuncture actually do?" *pg 72*
- "What can acupuncture not do?" *pg 74*

## Q. When should I think about getting an acupuncture treatment?

The "when" question is an easy one, so let's tackle that first. The answer is today. Seriously. If acupuncture can help you live your best life, then why would you wait?

But what I think you mean is "On what basis would I get an acupuncture treatment?" which is really a question of "why."

I think the answer to this is a dive into your priorities for yourself. Are you OK having a medical problem that you just deal with? Does it bother you that you will have to take a pill for something like cholesterol, blood sugar control, high blood pressure, pain, or digestive problems for the rest of your life? Do you think that it is easier to take anti-anxiety medications for your mental health support than to look into other options? If this describes you, then acupuncture is probably not a good solution for you.

Acupuncture looks at the root cause of all of the things that are bothering you and then works to solve the root cause so that all the branches of your mind, body, and emotions are "better." It helps to get you off of your medications—in collaboration with the clinician that prescribed them, of course. Yes, this is the case even for many of the medical problems for which you've been told you need medications indefinitely.

Acupuncture is extremely helpful in situations where the checking account of your health is tapped out and you need to dive into your savings account—like undergoing cancer treatment. The cancer itself is horrible. While my medical and surgical colleagues are always working to make it less so, the treatment is also horrible. Your savings account will likely be tapped into pretty significantly if you are undergoing cancer treatment. This is where acupuncture can support your ability to tolerate treatment and to recover from the cancer and the treatment. The fatigue, nausea, lack of sleep, nutritional support, feelings of hopelessness, grief or despair, and general strain on all rapidly-dividing cells in your body that result from many chemotherapy treatments are helped and abated by acupuncture. This is well-established in the medical literature.

The big stressors on Maslow's hierarchy will similarly tap into your savings account—job changes, death of a loved one (parent, spouse, child, or close friend), moving, etc. People are often very stressed about news events, political situations, neighborhood or community problems, religious issues, etc. For all of these situations, acupuncture can support your body, mind, and emotions as you navigate them.

For all of these reasons, including just being curious about it, please consider getting acupuncture today. Go on...

## SEE ALSO

- "How does an acupuncturist formulate a diagnosis and treatment plan?" *pg 56*
- "Can you use acupuncture as preventative medicine?" *pg 88*
- "What does acupuncture actually do?" *pg 72*
- "What can acupuncture not do?" *pg 74*

## Q. Does acupuncture treat pain?

Yes. The medical literature here is so vast and so solid that the Department of Defense, the Veterans Health Association, the Center for Medicare and Medicaid Services, and many other health-related organizations employ acupuncturists and/or cover the use of acupuncture for pain.

Acupuncture can treat pain that just came on (acute pain) and pain that has been around for a long time (chronic pain). It can treat sharp, stabbing, dull, achy, throbbing, intermittent, and/or constant pain. Pain with pins and needles, pain with numbness, pain with hot or cold sensations, and pain with searing sensations can all be treated with acupuncture.

Acupuncture has been adopted by physical therapists in the form of dry needling because it is so good at treating pain. Acupuncture is used as "trigger point therapy" because it is so good at treating pain.

When James Reston wrote his 1971 article on the front page of the New York Times, his amazement was that three acupuncture needles had been used to treat his pain after having his appendix removed emergently on a trip to China. He was amazed he didn't need anything else for pain after his surgery.

There are American studies that show acupuncture alone can be used instead of anesthesia to control pain during skin grafts, hysterectomy, neck surgeries, and abdominal surgery. Yes, you read that correctly. You can shave layers of someone's skin off and staple or sew it to another part of their body using only acupuncture to control the pain of that procedure.

In my clinical practice, there have been some pains that I have not been able to treat, so I don't want to be so emphatic that I mislead you into thinking that acupuncture can fix every kind of pain in every situation for every person. Pains from tumors that are rapidly growing, for example, can be lessened but do not go away. The tumor keeps growing, so it keeps making the situation worse. Pains that come from an anatomical problem like a broken bone or a ripped ligament can be made tolerable (or more tolerable), but the bone still needs to be set and the ligament addressed. Back or neck pains that result from ruptured discs or nerve impingement can be very difficult to treat with acupuncture alone. In my experience, I use acupuncture to make it tolerable while the person waits for surgery or I use acupuncture in conjunction with other integrative, collaborative approaches.

That said, yes, acupuncture is overall very, very good at treating pain.

---

### SEE ALSO

- "What is the history of acupuncture in the West?" *pg 159*
- "How long do the benefits of acupuncture last?" *pg 102*

---

## Q. What is the success rate of acupuncture?

I am including this question because it is commonly asked. However, for a book of this size, I simply cannot answer this very complicated question. Here is why.

## How conventional medicine measures success rate

Conventional medicine prides itself on being able to predict, with varying degrees of certainty, whether or not a person will do "well" with a procedure, medication, or intervention. It is able to establish these predictions because it has research money for investigating who will most benefit and who will not benefit from the intervention. That money comes from places like the National Institutes of Health, grant funding, drug companies, and device companies, all of whom are invested in finding the "best" outcomes for people. There are complicated algorithms, for example, for whether or not a partial or total knee replacement surgery is "indicated," based on your particular situation.

In the trials that establish the success rates of an intervention, a limited variety of factors are considered: your lifestyle, your gender, how serious the issue is, and related health conditions you might have or not have.

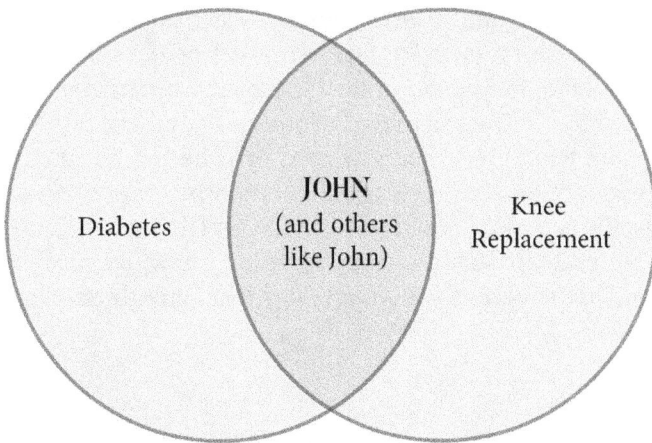

Most clinicians know—and can quote—the probability of a particular outcome for a given set of patients. To use the example above, if John needs a knee replacement surgery (the intervention) and has diabetes (a related health condition), the chances of him having a successful operation without complications are XX% (success rate).

But here's the thing, no clinician can tell you the success rate of conventional medicine overall. Those statistics are too vast and too complicated. If you'd like to learn a little more, please read on.

## What is not considered in calculating success rates

What is not generally considered in calculating those success rates—but is absolutely related—is a wide variety of less easily measured factors. Can John get access to transportation, medical services like home healthcare, and medical devices like crutches or a wheelchair? Does John have the time and financial ability to access physical or occupational therapy and other logistical support? Can he take the time off from work to get treated and does that put his job (and health insurance) at risk? Does John have financial stressors when he takes time off or does he get medical leave? Does he eat lots of fresh fruits and vegetables or highly processed food? Does he have friends and family or other means of support while he is being treated or if he has an unexpected consequence? Success rates are influenced by all of these things. Finally, the success is based on his provider (their skill, knowledge and ability), their staff and support team, the wider medical system, and, to be honest, the kind of day that all of those people are having.

Doing statistics on all of these factors would be very difficult because a person would have to create groups for each of these variables and then get enough people that need knee replacements and study them all. When you treat someone as an individual with unique health history, needs, and background, there are too many individual considerations. Each person in this scenario becomes too unique for statistics like success rate.

Do you see where I'm going here?

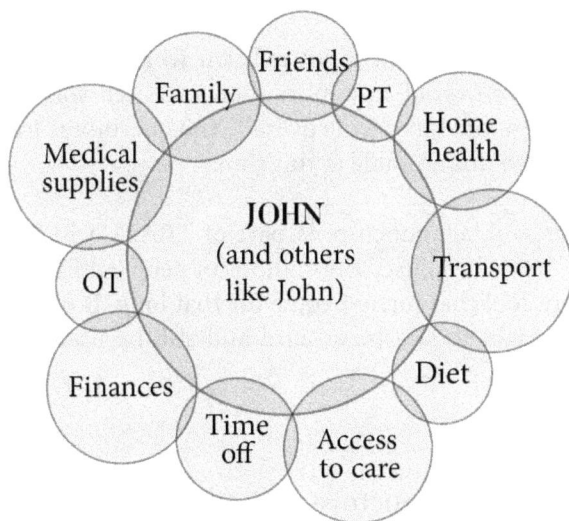

### How acupuncture is practiced

Acupuncture is contextual medicine. It treats you as an individual in the context of all of the things above. The fact that you are a person with diabetes who needs a knee replacement surgery is just a small part of the context of you as a whole person. If an acupuncturist treats John, Renee, and Shawna for diabetes and knee pain, the acupoints selected will be unique to each one because each one is a unique person.

This makes it complicated to do the same kind of research that is done in conventional medicine to measure success rates. Some acupuncture researchers have done studies like this, but they have to make the Venn diagram more similar to the first one. This takes some of the tailored treatment choices out of the research, which then skews the research results because acupuncture is not being done in the study in the same way it is done in "real life."

Because of all of this, I cannot tell you what the success rate is of acupuncture overall, any more than I can tell you the success rate of conventional medicine overall. The question is too big, too broad, and too unknowable at this time.

All of that said, acupuncture is part of TEAM, which is >2,500 years old. It has been used on millions of people during that time. You cannot fool that many people for that long. It must be doing something right to still be around and still be used and still be sought after.

## Q. Can I use acupuncture with other methods for my issues?

Yes, absolutely. There is no reason your other methods of treatment need to stop because you are receiving acupuncture treatment. By all means, see your massage therapist, your colon hydro-therapist, your cardiologist, your dietician, your Craniosacral practitioner, and your talk therapist. I've even had conversations with personal trainers and life coaches on behalf of patients.

Most acupuncturists recommend a collaborative approach to care and will gladly communicate openly and honestly with other practitioners caring for your medical, physical, and mental health.

My only request is that you not receive dry needling when you are receiving acupuncture. Dry needling is a subtype of acupuncture that is very vigorous and can be disruptive to the healing process stimulated by whole-body acupuncture treatments.

## SEE ALSO

- "Where do the needles go?" *pg 133*
- "Do the needles hurt?" *pg 114*
- "What is the difference between acupuncture and dry needling?" *pg 151*
- "Does acupuncture interfere with my other medical treatments?" *pg 119*
- "What other kinds of practitioners can use acupuncture needles?" *pg 149*
- "References" *pg 181*

# CHAPTER FOUR

# WHAT IS THE IDEAL TIMING BETWEEN MY ACUPUNCTURE TREATMENTS?

## Q. How quickly does acupuncture work?

This varies based on your overall health and how long the condition has been going on. It is also based, of course, on the skill of your practitioner.

Generally speaking, conditions that have been going on for a short time or are less severe respond more quickly to acupuncture. If your body has developed excruciating elbow pain from years and years of tennis, computer work, and rock climbing, it will take more time to get you out of pain than if you twisted your arm yesterday and are coming for treatment today.

That being said, I have had situations where someone is coming to me for severe abdominal pain that has been going on for years, and I resolved it in one treatment. In other situations, issues that I expected would take only a few treatments went on for a few months. This past week, someone with 6-8 hot flashes each night told me that after the second treatment, she had only 1 hot flash and slept better than she had in 6 months. When I was receiving acupuncture treatment for a similar condition, it took about 6 weeks for me to go from 8-12 hot flashes per night to none.

People typically feel a difference after one treatment of acupuncture. It might be small. The effects might not last 100% until your next treatment. But it is rare that a person doesn't feel something at each visit when receiving acupuncture from a qualified acupuncturist.

---

### SEE ALSO

- "How long do the benefits of acupuncture last?" *pg 102*

- "How do you know if acupuncture is working?" *pg 105*

- "How often do I have to go for treatment?" *pg 108*

---

## Q. How long do the benefits of acupuncture last?

I hate to say "it depends," but there is just not one quick answer for this question. It's like asking "How long do the effects of a medication last and how much do you have to take?" To answer the medication question, we have to give hundreds of people the same dose and then monitor the blood levels of the drug and the effects of the medication, plot it on a bell curve, and create dosing regimens. Those bell curves are always based on percentages, which means that some people will be in the middle "normal" range of the bell curve and some people will fall outside the normal ranges on the bell curve. The people who are not normal might need more or less medication than the people in the middle of the curve. It has to be tested and is part of the drug's approval process. The drug company also tested the dose and plotted a graph that shows where most of the people who took the drug had the desired effect. This is why some drugs are given at 10 mg and others at 100 mg. Some once a day and some four times a day. So knowing how a medication works is based on population statistics. It is not something that scientists automatically know based on its chemistry when a pharmaceutical drug is manufactured. You have to put the drug in human beings and test its pharmacokinetics.

Because acupuncture is a customized form of healthcare, it is inherently challenging to even find a group of people that are similar enough to form a cohesive cohort. You would then have to give all of the people in the cohort the same amount of acupuncture at the same points, get them to give constant feedback on exactly when their issue resolved (This is much harder than you think because people don't often notice the absence of pain. They generally only notice when it is there.), have people who can plot and analyze all the data (Also much harder than it sounds.), and develop a graph that defines "normal" and establishes standard deviations from normal. You would have to do that with every kind of problem that a group of people could possibly have. Soooo...this is not impossible, but close.

Having said all that, very, very generally speaking, the effects of an acupuncture last for a few hours to days after the first treatment, and then a little bit longer after the next treatment, and then a little bit longer after the next treatment, and on like that until your issue is resolved or tolerable. But it depends on whether you are in the middle or edges of the bell curve, whether your practitioner is in the middle or the edges of bell curve for their skill level for your particular problem, whether your problem is new or old, whether you are eating good food and exercising and sleeping and taking care of yourself, whether you have the capacity to do the stretches or take the herbs or do the things your practitioner asks you to do, and on a whole lot of other things.

This might sound like a bunch of excuses. I get that. Instead, this is, in my experience, because your body develops habits that contribute to—or are in reaction to—the reasons you might seek treatment. You are a complex person with a unique history, and your health issues are rarely straight forward.

For example, you might develop a slight limp because you twisted your ankle. This results in torque in your knee when you walk, and over time, a feeling of discomfort in your hip and lower back. If you come in to be treated for the lower back pain, I'm not doing you any favors to just focus on your back. Your whole leg needs to be addressed from your hip to your ankle. You're likely going to continue to walk every day while I'm trying to do work on your leg for an hour once a week, so you are "undoing" what I am doing with the treatments for a time while we are retraining your body to not have the habit of walking with a limp. All of this takes time, and it's hard to predict exactly when and how much your back will feel better as we are working on your back AND all the other relevant issues influencing how your back feels.

Working in this way is also preventing you from further wear and tear on joints that you are moving in a suboptimal way from the time that we start fixing your body mechanics until the day that you are no longer with us. From this perspective and in this kind of context, the benefits of acupuncture would last the rest of your life.

If you come to see me for shoulder pain that is from getting out of the car in a funny way a few days ago—assuming you haven't ripped or broken something—the benefits of acupuncture would typically last a few days in the beginning and then longer and longer with subsequent treatments until you don't need me anymore. Short-term injuries or pains can be fixed quickly, and results typically last for long periods of time. Conversely and for reasons that I hope are obvious to you now, longer term problems take longer for you to feel better, longer for you to feel completely better between treatments, and longer for you to not need additional treatments.

---

### SEE ALSO

- "How quickly does acupuncture work?" *pg 101*
- "How long do the benefits of acupuncture last?" *pg 102*
- "How do you know if acupuncture is working?" *pg 105*
- "How often do I have to go for treatment?" *pg 108*

---

## Q. How do you know if acupuncture is working?

Acupuncture is working if you feel better. That might mean your pain is lessened. That might mean that your digestion is working better, and you are less bloated or gassy or gurgley. That might mean that you are sleeping more soundly, find it easier to fall asleep, and feel more rested when you get up. That might mean your emotions are less wonky, and you feel calmer and more empowered in your life. That might mean your energy is better and you have more patience with your kids and spouse because you don't feel like you're falling apart at the seams.

Some acupuncturists like to use numerical scales or questionnaires to quantify progress because we humans tend to forget how bad it actually was 3 months or 6 months or 12 months ago. These tools help to remind us with objective data about what is getting better and how much...and what still needs to be addressed.

Even if you are coming only for pain, there are often other concomitant problems that you have been told by conventional medicine to "just live with." Those things often start to get better at the same time I am treating your pain.

As just one example, I had a 58-year-old patient I was treating for digestive issues. She had cancer in her neck when she was 17 years old, and had received surgery and radiation to that area. She was deaf in her right ear as a consequence. I treated her digestive issues, and she noticed that her hearing was improving. She even had it tested professionally with an audiologist, and after 40+ years of not being able to hear, working on her as a whole person in the context of TEAM not only fixed her primary digestive concerns, but it also made a difference with issues we were not specifically intending to treat. We did a happy dance together when we realized she was getting her hearing back, and it gave me yet another lesson in appreciation and respect for the power of TEAM.

I also know acupuncture is working because I practice a style of acupuncture that is largely Japanese in origin. In this style, I might push on a particular spot on your belly (Ren 12) to see if it is tender, indicating that there is some stagnant Qi that needs to be moved. If it is tender, I might place an acupuncture needle in your leg at an acupoint that I know releases that stagnant Qi (ST 36). After I feel the Qi arrive under my needle tip, I would come back and check that belly spot again to see if it is still tender. If it is still tender, I know I need to add some additional acupoints and/ or tweak the placement of the needle in your leg. If it is not tender, we both know acupuncture is working because the stagnation that was causing that tender spot before has been removed by the insertion of the acupuncture needle (in a totally different area of your body than the tender spot!). The needle in your leg acupoint has unblocked the traffic jam in your whole-body meridian highway system and is letting things flow more freely all the way up into your abdomen.

I began to trust acupuncture because I know that there are no nerve or blood vessel pathways that connect these two points (and many other similar tender-release-double check points). The change has to be happening through some other communication pathway. Based on the functions of the relationships between the tender point and the needled point, I think it's the meridian pathway. The effects are reproducible with those points in patient after patient after patient. And the patient—not just the practitioner—experiences the change in how they feel from one second to the next. It was tender a few seconds ago. I placed a needle. Now it is not tender anymore. It's pretty convincing stuff once you feel it in your own body. All of that tells me acupuncture is working.

Finally, you know it is working because of the second-to-second changes that I can elicit in your pulse or tongue when I place the needles. I love to do this with the medical students that I have in clinic sometimes; I have them feel the person's pulses as I am doing the needling. As I feel the arrival of Qi under the tip of my acupuncture needle, I will direct the student's attention to the corresponding pulse that they are feeling with their left ring finger or right index finger. I tell them a second before the pulse will change, and then their eyes get really big with shock when they feel the pulse jump up under their finger. Similarly, the patient's tongue changes before and after treatment, and the students are consistently amazed when I point out the differences.

So while it is admittedly challenging to know exactly when acupuncture starts working, there are lots of ways to know that it does.

## SEE ALSO

- "What is Qi?" *pg 20*
- "How quickly does acupuncture work?" *pg 101*

- "How long do the benefits of acupuncture last?" *pg 102*
- "How often do I have to go for treatment?" *pg 108*
- "Why does the acupuncturist want to see my tongue and feel my wrists?" *pg 130*

## Q. How often do I have to go for treatment?

As discussed, you should feel better after the first treatment and that "feeling better feeling" will generally last for 1-3 days, after which you will start feeling like you felt before. Your body has developed the habit of feeling or behaving that way (having pain or not sleeping well or whatever it is) for a reason. Acupuncture has to have time to retrain your body to behave differently.

I try to time a second treatment soon after the first so that I can again launch you in the direction of the "feeling better feeling." After a few treatments the effects last longer and longer until they are, hopefully, resolved or tolerable.

So treatments should be more frequent in the beginning (1-2x/ week on average). After you start to feel better and the effects last longer, you come once a week, then every 10-14 days, and so on until you stop coming or come in "as needed."

This is very similar to other medical therapies like talk therapy or physical therapy. If you are in an acute emotional state, you might need to speak to your therapist more than once a week. As you feel better, you cut back to once a week and then slowly every other week or once a month. If you feel really great, you might stop going altogether or you might continue because you like knowing that you have a professional's ear once a month to help you work through challenges in your life.

Similarly, you might go to PT several times a week after a shoulder surgery and then decrease the frequency of your appointments as your shoulder feels better and you gain function back.

In my practice, the end goal of treatment is always that you don't need me anymore. I want you to graduate from needing me and move into the phase of "I just feel so good when I come for a treatment that I'd like to come regularly as preventative medicine or to keep my symptoms in check at the level where they are now." Although I will miss seeing you more often, this is a wonderful phase where we can start preventing problems from coming up for you instead of having to react to problems that have already arisen. It makes me sad to say goodbye, but it is beyond gratifying to facilitate a person's healing and send them off into the world feeling fabulous. I just love it.

## SEE ALSO

- "How quickly does acupuncture work?" *pg 101*
- "How long do the benefits of acupuncture last?" *pg 102*
- "How do you know if acupuncture is working?" *pg 105*
- "Can you use acupuncture as preventative medicine?" *pg 88*

# CHAPTER FIVE

# WHAT ARE THE SIDE EFFECTS AND RISKS OF ACUPUNCTURE?

## Q. Is acupuncture safe? What are the risks of acupuncture?

Yes, acupuncture is safe and has low risks, but the risk is not zero. The risk of having anything seriously bad happen to you when getting an acupuncture treatment is less than the risk of having something seriously bad happen to you during a routine colonoscopy. I'm picking this procedure to compare acupuncture to because it is something that most people have to have at some point (or multiple points) in their lives and because we tend to think about it as a low-risk procedure.

You're probably thinking, "what on earth can happen when I'm getting a colonoscopy?" Well, the doctor can perforate your colon—make a hole in it—which means you need to have emergency surgery to create a colostomy bag on your belly while that perforation hole heals. Later on, you need another surgery to close off the colostomy hole. You can have bleeding, infections, damage to the muscles and the sphincters, and a myriad of other things. So you can see that there are definitely risks involved, not even counting the risks of anesthesia and drug reactions. Yet, we consider it a pretty safe procedure, as procedures go.

The minor risks of acupuncture are things like small bruises or bleeding where the acupuncture needles are inserted. "Bleeding" here means a few drops of blood easily stopped by gentle pressure with a cotton ball after the needle is removed. I try to prevent that by using very tiny needles (0.14 to 0.2 mm in diameter, which is a little bit bigger than the diameter of the hair on your head and much smaller than needles used when they draw blood) and placing them superficially into the skin—about 2-4 mm deep. This applies to about 90% of the acupoints I use. Occasionally, however, I need to go deeper.

The risks of going deeper with acupuncture needles are that they can go into a structure and create a tiny hole. This is not a problem in tissues like muscles, generally speaking, but it's less great in arteries or veins, which would result in bigger bruises or collections of blood (like a hematoma). However, studies have shown that this is extremely rare even in people who are on blood thinners or anti-clotting medications.

Making tiny holes can also be problematic in bowels or lungs. In fact, making a tiny hole in the lung that causes the lung to collapse—a pneumothorax—is a known risk of acupuncture. But it is very, very rare. You would know this had happened during the treatment because you would feel short of breath or have some pain in your chest when you are breathing. You are at an increased risk of this happening if you are a smoker or if you are a tall, thin person. (Tall, thin people have long lung spaces and don't have much muscle between their skin and their lung spaces.)

The needles are sterile and used only once before placing them in a sharps container for disposal. Acupuncturists have to complete a certificate indicating extensive training in "clean needle technique" before they can take their board exams. However, there is still a small risk of infection.

Practitioners are at a slightly increased risk of a needle stick—pricking themselves with an acupuncture needle when they are placing or removing needles. I mention it for completeness because it is a known risk, but the practitioner pricking themselves accidentally is not a risk to you as the patient—only to them.

There is a small risk of pain at the site of the needle entry. That pain usually goes away in a few seconds. If it continues, the needle may be too close to a nerve. Just inform the acupuncturist to adjust the needle so it does not continue to be painful.

Finally, there are limited reports of nausea, sweating, or other autonomic responses. For example, the needles can sometimes make you feel a little "needle drunk," which means you might feel a little dizzy, woozy, or "off." This is most common when you haven't eaten anything or are dehydrated before coming in for a treatment. I always recommend to my patients that they drink some water and eat meals or snacks on days when they are having a treatment for this reason.

While I have given you a long list of issues that can happen with acupuncture treatment with the intention of being as comprehensive as possible, please let me say again that the risk of any of these things happening is very low. It's not zero, but it's very low.

## SEE ALSO

- "Does acupuncture interfere with my other medical treatments?" *pg 119*
- "What other kinds of practitioners can use acupuncture needles?" *pg 149*
- "References" *pg 181*

## Q. Do the needles hurt?

Acupuncture needles are not like the needles we use to draw blood. Phlebotomy needles are hollow and have a beveled, cutting end on them. They are designed to cut through your skin and cut into your blood vessel to pull out blood. This cutting action is what hurts.

Having an injection is similarly painful because the needle point is designed for cutting and also because the substance being injected is not the same acid/base balance (pH) as your body tissues. This causes a burning sensation as the substance is injected and an inflammatory reaction afterwards. Inflammation causes pain.

Acupuncture needles are solid and have a slightly rounded tip on them. They are designed to push tissue out of the way—to insert into the tissue without cutting it. As such, they are designed to cause minimal discomfort.

Most acupuncturists use a needle introducer—a small guide tube that holds the acupuncture needle. This introducer serves two purposes. It keeps the tip of the needle sterile. The acupuncturist only touches the handle of the needle, keeping the tip of the needle clean.

The other purpose of the tube is that the acupuncturist pushes the introducer slightly onto the skin. This activates the pressure sensors in your skin. When the pressure sensors are activated, they suppress the local pain receptors from firing. So the introducer has a "numbing" function on the surrounding pain receptors, making the needle less painful as it goes into the skin. This is similar to rubbing your elbow after you hit it on the door. You're activating the pressure sensors in the area, which works to dull the pain signals.

I practiced on myself for years to achieve a painless needling technique which works for my patients about 95-99% of the time. In other words, if I needle 10 people a day in 10 places (100 sites total), 1-5 of those needles will hurt for a few seconds on average. Those are good odds.

One of the reasons for those little zings of discomfort is that you do have small nerves distributed all throughout your skin. Sometimes I accidentally touch them with the tip of my needle. There is no anatomical map for the tiny nerves—only for the big ones—so it is not possible to predict exactly where they are and prevent this from happening on occasion. To fix this, I just move the needle so it is not touching the nerve.

Needles that are placed into sites where the skin is very thin there is very little padding from fat or muscles (top of the feet, fingers and toes, back of the hand, etc.) are similarly more likely to be painful. However, that pain should only last a second or two. If it lasts longer, simply ask the acupuncturist to adjust the needle.

I find that when women are on their period, the hormone fluctuations make acupuncture a bit more painful during that week. I also find that some people are just a little more sensitive than others. For menstruating women and particularly sensitive people, I use even smaller needles or needles that have a silicone coating that makes them even more slippery and less likely to be painful. If someone is very, very sensitive, we just use some other tool (lasers, moxa, teshin, or gua sha) instead of needles.

Finally, some practitioners look for people to experience an achy, warm feeling at the site of the acupuncture needles. This is called the "de Qi" (which translates as "the Qi" so that sentence reads "the the Qi"—oh well) sensation at the acupoint. It feels achy or warm in the same way that rubbing a sore muscle hurts a little bit but also feels good. That sore muscle is sore because it has been overused or injured in some way. From a TEAM perspective, the soreness indicates stagnation or pooling, which is the opposite of free-flowing Qi (Yang). The *de Qi* sensation indicates we acupuncturists have found a place of stagnation and are moving it strongly with acupuncture needling and related techniques.

Some people really like the *de Qi* sensation when they receive acupuncture, but for other people it is too strong. If this is not a sensation that you enjoy, simply ask the acupuncturist to make the needling less intense or strong for you or look for a practitioner who is able to needle with Japanese style acupuncture, which is more gentle and relies less on achieving *de Qi*.

## SEE ALSO

- "How does the thought theory of acupuncture differ from conventional medicine?" *pg 163*
- "What is the history of acupuncture in the West?" *pg 159*
- "What other kinds of things can an acupuncturist do?" *pg 145*
- "Is acupuncture safe? What are the risks of acupuncture?" *pg 111*

## Q. Can I have acupuncture even though I'm on a blood thinner or anti-clotting medication?

Yes, it is generally safe for you to receive acupuncture even when you are on a blood thinner or anti-clotting medicine. "Coagulation" is the process of blood congealing to make a clot. "Anticoagulation" refers to medicines or processes that prevent that from happening.

The medical literature shows that people on anticoagulants do not have a significantly increased risk of minor bleeding like bruises or of more serious bleeding like hematomas. (A hematoma is an abnormal collection of blood between the tissues that is bigger than a bruise.)

In one study that looked at 384 patients receiving anticoagulant medicines, the researchers found one moderate bleeding event in 3,974 treatments, making a complication rate of 0.003%. That moderate bleeding event was a small hematoma that was treated by stopping the anticoagulant medicine warfarin and giving vitamin K to reverse the effects of warfarin.

Blood spot bleeding (a tiny drop or two of blood when the acupuncture needle is removed) was seen in 51 out of 350 treatments (14.6%) in another study. No bleeding was reported in two studies involving 74 anticoagulated patients.

In another large study, micro bleeding (bleeding at the skin that stopped within 30 seconds with light pressure), slight bruising and fatigue were the only side effects reported in patients anti-coagulated with warfarin and having a high PT INR (a measure of how anti coagulated a person is).

There are many more studies than I am referencing here, but I hope that this abbreviated list shows you that acupuncture is generally safe for people who are taking anticoagulant medicines.

## SEE ALSO

- "Is acupuncture safe? What are the risks of acupuncture?" *pg 111*
- "Is acupuncture safe for children? For physically challenged people? For elderly people?" *pg 121*
- "References" *pg 181*

## Q. Does acupuncture cause scarring?

I can theoretically see that this could happen. However, I have never seen it happen and have not read about it happening in the medical literature either before in my routine reviews of the literature or now in preparation for writing this book. I have never heard of it happening in a case report, class, conference, or continuing education course I have attended.

Because acupuncture needles are very, very thin, it is unlikely they would cause an injury to the skin so large that it would even scab, much less scar. However, the needles do go into the skin, and so it is always a theoretical possibility that a small scab and scar could form. Bodies are unpredictable that way.

Moxibustion (or "moxa"), which is a practice of using an herb on the skin and smoldering the herb to penetrate the skin with the healing oils and heat from the herb, has been known to create scars from small burns. Historically speaking, moxa that was intended to create scarring was used for treatment of chronic or deep problems, but this is not a common practice currently in the US.

People who have diabetes or other problems which might compromise the sensation they have in their skin are at a slightly increased risk of developing a scar from use of moxibustion, but that risk—even in diabetics—is very low.

### SEE ALSO

• "Is acupuncture safe? What are the risks of acupuncture?" *pg 111*

## Q. Does acupuncture interfere with my other medical treatments?

### *Cancer Treatment*

Acupuncture is an increasingly common adjunct for people undergoing cancer treatment, and many large cancer treatment centers employ acupuncturists. An acupuncturist needs to stay away from chemotherapy ports, maintain very clean acupoints to diminish any risk of infection, and be cautious about "overstimulating" someone who is depleted. But acupuncture does not interfere with cancer treatment. In fact, it is often very helpful in supporting a person going through chemotherapy, radiation, or surgery for cancer.

Because herbs can interfere with cancer treatment regimens, I do not prescribe herbal medicines without discussing it with the person and with a person's oncologists to make sure that 1.) the patient is not caught in a disagreement or miscommunication between practitioners and 2.) everyone is on the same page about any potential benefits, side effects, or interactions.

### *Medications*

Acupuncture does not interfere with medications except to say that people often don't need as many medications after they come for acupuncture. For example, people's blood pressure goes down with acupuncture therapy, so they need less high blood pressure or diuretic medications. They might need fewer acid blockers because their heartburn symptoms improve or resolve. Their blood sugar is better controlled, so they need less insulin support or diabetes medications. This is not great for the drug companies, but most people are pretty happy about needing to take fewer pills. In my practice, I see over and over again that we are able to communicate with the person prescribing the medication and cut back or wean off of many medications.

As above, it is important that the licensed acupuncturist know about all pharmaceutical medicines and supplements a person is taking so that they can guard against any side effects if they prescribe herbal medicines.

## *Physical Therapy*

While your PT might employ a technique called "dry needling" that is a simplistic, limited subtype of acupuncture, it is not the same as getting acupuncture from a licensed acupuncturist. Getting acupuncture does not interfere with dry needling or other physical therapy. However, getting dry needling might detract from your acupuncture treatments because it is much more aggressive and less sophisticated than comprehensive, whole-person acupuncture performed by a fully-trained acupuncturist.

### SEE ALSO

- "What other kinds of practitioners can use acupuncture needles?" *pg 149*
- "Do the needles hurt?" *pg 114*
- "Can I use acupuncture with other methods for my issues?" *pg 98*
- "What is the difference between acupuncture and dry needling?" *pg 151*
- "References" *pg 181*

## Q. Is acupuncture safe for children? For physically challenged people? For elderly people?

### *Children*

In my practice, I do acupuncture for children around two years old and older. Younger than that, I use another tool that presses on the acupoint called a "teshin" or a skin scraping tool called a "gua sha" tool. I try to use the absolute fewest number of needles possible and give the child a chance to look at the needles if they want to ahead of time. I talk the child through what will happen so that they feel safe and don't worry about me sneaking up on them. I often use counting or deep breathing to help distract the child, and I tell them they can squeeze my arm as hard as they want to as I'm putting the needle in. After the first needle—when they realize that it really doesn't hurt nearly as much as getting a shot (if they feel it at all)—they generally don't mind the acupuncture treatments and tend to look forward to them as much as adults do.

### *Physically challenged people*

For physically challenged people, I make sure I accommodate them by treating them in a position that is maximally comfortable, working with chronic problems gently and slowly, and by knowing lots of options to treat the same problem.

For example, if a person doesn't have a left arm and I would normally use the left arm to treat their primary concerns, I need to know other acupoints that can treat that issue. If a person has a lot of spastic, unpredictable movements in their legs, I need to pick acupoints on the upper parts of the body.

For mentally challenged people, obtaining consent is the first issue. If necessary, it needs to be done through the medical power of attorney, involving the patient as much as possible. For people who do not fully understand what is happening to them, I do not leave them unattended in the treatment room with needles in their bodies for safety reasons. This is no different than accommodating the needs of any other patient in my practice and tailoring my conversations and treatment to meet their needs.

## Elderly people

Older people respond very well to acupuncture treatment, and many of my elderly patients report feeling "better than they have in years" after treatment. In my practice, I tend to be gentler with needling depth/intensity and use fewer needles in elderly patients, recognizing that as we age the skin can become thinner and this increases the chances of causing a little bit of pain when the needle is inserted into the acupoint. As previously discussed, even though many elderly people are on medications like blood thinners, they can still safely receive acupuncture treatment.

### SEE ALSO

- "Is acupuncture safe? What are the risks of acupuncture?" *pg 111*
- "Do the needles hurt?" *pg 114*
- "Can I have acupuncture even though I'm on a blood thinner or anti-clotting medication?" *pg 116*
- "References" *pg 181*

## Q. Does acupuncture cause infections?

It is very, very rare for acupuncture to cause an infection. People who have a compromised immune system, are taking immune suppressing medications like steroids or chemotherapy agents, or have diabetes have a slightly increased risk of developing an infection for any reason, which includes receiving acupuncture.

Acupuncture needles are packaged in sterile packaging. They are generally placed in the skin using a guide tube or introducer that is also packed in sterile packaging or cleaned regularly with alcohol. The needles are used only one time and then disposed of in sharps containers. If the needle tip is accidentally touched by the acupuncturist or brushes up against any other surface (the bed, sheets, table, etc.), it is disposed of without using it.

As a part of their licensure, acupuncturists must take a comprehensive course and pass an exam in "clean needle technique." This course covers the handling of acupuncture needles and other tools commonly used in acupuncture. An acupuncturist cannot sit for their national board exams (NCCAOM exams) without completing this course.

While the risk is not zero, the risk of infection is extremely small because of all of this cleanliness training, attention to detail, and sterile tools.

### SEE ALSO

- "Do acupuncturists take board exams?" *pg 139*
- "Is acupuncture safe? What are the risks of acupuncture?" *pg 111*
- "What are acupuncture needles made of?" *pg 134*

# CHAPTER SIX

# WHAT ARE THE LOGISTICS OF ACUPUNCTURE TREATMENT?

## Q. What should I expect at a treatment?

### Examination

When you arrive, the acupuncturist will take your medical history and do a physical exam. In addition to any needed conventional medical physical exam tests, the acupuncturist will feel your pulses with three fingers at your wrists and want to look at your tongue. The pulses and tongue evaluations give us a sense of how your organ systems are working together and which are depleted or excessive. Many acupuncturists use changes in the pulses and/or tongue to guide treatment as both can change when acupoints are stimulated.

### Treatment

The acupuncturist will explain the treatment to you and obtain your informed consent. You will lay down in a comfortable position—commonly on a massage table—or sit in a reclined chair if you are in a community acupuncture clinic. It is helpful to wear loosely fitting clothing that exposes your arms up to your elbows and your legs up to your knees. Forearms and lower legs are the areas an acupuncturist will generally need to access for treatment. In some cases they might also want to access your abdomen, upper chest, and/or back. If that is the case, you will change into a gown and/or be draped with a sheet for modesty.

The acupuncturist will place the needles and then let you rest with the needles in place for a time, around 20-40 minutes on average. Often there is soft music playing and a heat lamp on a part of your body or heat coming from the bed. Many people fall asleep during the treatment. The acupuncturist might also use other techniques during treatment.

### After treatment

After the treatment is over, the acupuncturist or their assistant will remove the needles and perform a needle count to make sure they have removed all of them.

The acupuncturist will work with you to create a treatment schedule. They might also recommend dietary changes, herbal medicines, lifestyle modifications, or supplements to support your treatment.

### SEE ALSO

- "What other kinds of things can an acupuncturist do?" *pg 145*

# Q. How should I prepare for an appointment?

## *Clothing choices*

Most acupuncturists will treat you with your clothing on, but some will ask you to change into a gown. If you are being treated with your clothing on, it is helpful to wear loose fitting clothes that allow exposure up to your elbows and up to your knees. These are the most common areas that the acupuncturist will use for needle placement. The acupuncturist might also want to access your abdomen or upper chest near your collarbones, so wearing a two-piece top and bottom instead of a single dress or bodysuit is generally preferred.

Try to wear clothing that allows the acupuncturist to access the area on your body where you want treatment. For example, if you are having shoulder pain, wear clothing that allows the acupuncturist to access your shoulder—a tank top instead of a turtleneck sweater, for example. Similarly, if you are coming for back or neck pain, the acupuncturist might need to access your back. In that case, it is helpful to wear a bra that opens to the back (and not a sports bra), so that your entire back is accessible.

If you have long hair, consider wearing your hair up or bringing a hair tie so that the acupuncturist can clearly view your neck and shoulders during treatment.

## *Time*

Allowing time to take a breath before and after your appointment supports the healing that happens during the appointment. If you are in fight/flight/freeze/fawn mode and your sympathetic nervous system is on high alert when you come in, your acupuncturist first has to help calm your nervous system down so that your body is ready to do housekeeping functions like healing, remodeling, digesting, and "cleaning house."

Additionally, if you are coming in for a "rest and digest" parasympathetic nervous system function like GI issues, sleep problems, difficulty with sexual function or hormones, and/or pain, your parasympathetic system has to be "in charge" before you can start healing the gut, endocrine system, nervous system, or places of injury.

This doesn't mean that you can't come for acupuncture until you are stress free of course—no one is stress free!—but one small way that you can facilitate your healing is by giving yourself the gift of not rushing in and not rushing out. Give yourself time to arrive and a few minutes before you go. Take a breath. Help yourself heal.

## *Nourishment*

One of my acupuncture teachers used to say that one of the best compliments that someone's body can give you is that their Stomach starts gurgling when you begin treating them. This is because the Stomach is the place where food begins to be turned into nourishment or "Gu Qi." Acupuncture moves Qi around in the body. So it is helpful to HAVE Qi so that there is Qi to actually move.

What I am getting at is that you should eat something before you come for a treatment. Don't starve yourself. Drink some water. Eat some food. Have some nourishment to work with. Starving yourself means you are coming to a pottery class but you left your clay at home—it makes it very hard to create something.

Drinking alcohol and using recreational drugs (including medical cannabis) is not ideal the day before and the day of treatment. This is because it manipulates your brain and/or body's chemistry. If you are already in a manipulated state when you come to your acupuncturist to be evaluated, it gives your clinician misinformation and impairs their ability to evaluate you accurately in your actual native state. This makes it harder to treat you effectively. Using those substances after treatment similarly disrupts the healing that has been stimulated by the acupuncture needles. I would not recommend it.

## Mental preparation

Sometimes people feel very anxious about receiving acupuncture. If this is the case for you, getting in touch with why you are feeling anxious can help your acupuncturist work with you to dissipate those anxious feelings.

If you are worried about the needles themselves, it can help to see a needle and touch it before your treatment. If it is a sense of not knowing what is coming or being worried about being surprised, ask your acupuncturist to talk you through what they are doing as they are working—to narrate out loud their thinking as they are picking points (and maybe why they are picking them).

If your anxiety about the needles is just too much, ask your acupuncturist if they can use other modalities that are not needles to treat you like cupping, tui na, Qi gong, gua sha, and other modalities. Acupuncturists can also use non-needle tools to stimulate the points such as moxibustion, cold light lasers, or a teshin.

In short, don't be afraid to bring up your concerns or questions with your practitioner. Despite its name, acupuncture is not only about needles: there are lots of other options.

## SEE ALSO

- "What other kinds of things can an acupuncturist do?" *pg 145*
- "Where do the needles go?" *pg 133*
- "Do the needles hurt?" *pg 114*

## Q. Why does the acupuncturist want to see my tongue and feel my wrists?

Just like going to a conventional doctor involves listening to your heart and lungs to get a sense of how well those organs are working or tapping on your reflexes to see how well your brain and nervous system are working, acupuncturists use observation, listening, smelling and palpation techniques to learn how well your body is functioning in the context of TEAM. We will go over the two main ones here.

### Tongue diagnosis

The body of your tongue is a microsystem of the main TEAM organs. Imagine that the tip of the tongue is facing up on a piece of paper and the back of the tongue is the bottom of the paper. Just like your mind is in the upper part of your body, the tip of your tongue at the top of the page reflects your "Shen" or emotional state of being, but in TEAM this is housed in the Heart. So the tip also reflects the Heart. If the tip is very red compared to the rest of the tongue, the acupuncturist might ask you about how well you are sleeping, if you feel anxious, or if you are feeling overheated (like having hot flashes) because the red heat is rising up to the top of your body and irritating your mind or your ability to relax.

The first part under the tip is the reflection site of the Lungs: they surround the Heart and are in the upper part of the body. Breast disease and chest issues also show up in this area.

The Liver and Gallbladder areas are on the sides of the tongue and the Spleen and Stomach areas are in the middle of the tongue. Quivering, puffiness, dusky coloring, and coating are all important parts of tongue diagnosis for these organs.

The acupuncturist will look at the base of your tongue to evaluate your Kidneys, Urinary Bladder and Intestines, which are located lower down on your body and so are at the bottom/base of your tongue. If you are having a hard time eliminating wastes, for example, the coat on your tongue might have a thick greasy appearance in this area.

By looking at cracks, color, coating, vessels under the tongue, and other signs, the acupuncturist gets a sense of your internal organs and how they are working together...or not.

### Pulse diagnosis

There are 12 primary organs in TEAM, just like there are 12 meridians. Twelve organs reflect to three locations on two wrists at two depths (3 x 2 x 2 = 12 pulses). The acupuncturist will place three fingers on each wrist and push their fingers against your pulses with varying pressure to identify characteristics of your pulse corresponding to each organ.[2]

---

2   *There are actually three depths to the pulse, but the organs correspond to only two of those three depths. Other practitioners consider the three depths of the pulse to be related to Qi, Blood and organs.*

This gets pretty complicated because there are 29 pulses described in TEAM, named by such descriptors as "soggy pulse" or "scattered pulse." It gets even more complicated because you can feel these different pulse characteristics in each of the 12 sites. It is a lot to concentrate on at once. This is why most acupuncturists close their eyes and don't talk while doing this. It is called "listening" to the pulse because of the intensity of concentration it requires. Many acupuncturists feel first one wrist and then the other rather than trying to feel them both at the same time.

## Other physical examination findings

I will tell you a secret that the acupuncturist is also using sound, smell, and taste to make diagnoses about you when you visit them. For example, frequent sighing is usually an indication that a person has Liver Qi stagnation, and constant laughing is a Heart Shen imbalance. If the person describes problems with bad breath, the acupuncturist might begin to think about Stomach Heat. If they describe a craving for salty snacks, the acupuncturist might question them about Water-related issues like back or knee pain, kidney stones, difficulty urinating or holding urine, or being "bone tired."

Pulse and tongue diagnosis are foundational to the acupuncturist understanding how you are and formulating your treatment plan.

### SEE ALSO

- "What Are the Foundational Concepts of Acupuncture?" *pg 13*
- "How do you know if acupuncture is working?" *pg 105*

# Q. Where do the needles go?

There are ~361 acupuncture points along the main highway system or meridians. There are more acupuncture points along the ancillary or "extraordinary" meridians. There are points along the meridians that correspond to Yin and Yang, Qi and Blood/Xue, and each of the organs in the system. There are points that are not on any meridians at all, and there are points in microsystems like the abdomen, hand, scalp, and face. The needles can go in any of those 2,000+ places.

They can also go in knots in your muscles or in achy, painful points on other parts of your body. These are called "Ah Shi" points—meaning "ouchy places"—and are the basis of trigger point needling and dry needling.

In some forms of acupuncture, reflection sites might be used. For example, the hand reflects to the head, the wrist to the neck, the forearm to the back (with the upper back being near the wrist and the lower back being near the elbow). Similarly the foot reflects to the head, the ankle to the neck, and the leg to the back (with the upper back toward the ankle and the lower back near the knee). There are maps for the entire body on the microsystems mentioned above. So if I am treating a headache, I might place needles in the head, the hand and the foot, since all reflect to the head.

If someone comes in with neck pain, I can put needles into their neck, but I don't have to. I can work with points that are on that same channel but not on the neck, which opens the traffic pattern of Qi in that meridian highway. I can use the wrists and ankles and places on the abdomen, hand, scalp, and face.

You're of course welcome to ask your acupuncturist why they are putting needles where they are—there is always a reason. But don't think that they have to stick you with needles in a place where it hurts or where the organ lives that is causing the issues for you.

Also, don't be surprised if you come in for a digestive issue, and the needles are placed in your arms and legs. The communication pathways are complex—like a highway map. There are many ways to select the path from "A" to "B."

---

**SEE ALSO**

- "How many acupuncture points are there?" *pg 66*
- "How does the acupuncturist pick which acupoints to use?" *pg 69*
- "What other kinds of practitioners can use acupuncture needles?" *pg 149*
- "What is the difference between acupuncture and dry needling?" *pg 151*

---

## Q. What are acupuncture needles made of?

Almost all of the acupuncture needles in use today in the United States are made of surgical stainless steel and are in sterile packaging. Acupuncturists touch the handles only and keep the needle tips (the part that actually goes into your body) sterile.

There are some clinicians that are using precious metals like gold or silver for acupuncture, but this is very rare. As you can imagine, doing that is pricey and so an acupuncturist would not "sneak" these needles without asking your permission to do so—and likely charging you extra.

If you are concerned about this, you can simply ask them to show you the packaging of the needles they are using. The packaging describes the type of metal used and has expiration dates for the sterility of the needles.

### SEE ALSO

- "Does acupuncture cause infections?" *pg 123*

# CHAPTER SEVEN

# WHO PRACTICES ACUPUNCTURE AND HOW ARE THEY TRAINED?

## Q. How are acupuncturists trained?

Acupuncturists must have at least 90 hours of undergraduate credits to enter professional school. After obtaining the required undergraduate credits, there are multiple routes of training in acupuncture schools.

The first is to earn a master's level degree or certificate. This consists of approximately 3-4 years of training and includes studies of biomedical sciences (anatomy, physiology, pathology, laboratory testing and radiographic studies, pharmacology, etc.), traditional East Asian medical theory (Zang Fu, five phases, organ and channel relationships, etc.), Chinese dietetics and food-based therapies, acupuncture (point locations, channels, and functions), ancillary techniques (tui na, gua sha, cupping, moxibustion, etc.), and mind-body techniques (Qi Gong, Tai Chi).

Most master's programs require at least an introductory course to herbal medicine. Herbal medicine coursework can be continued by the student and includes at least one year of single herbs and one year of herbal formulations (multiple herbs together). In order to sit for the NCCAOM board examination on herbal medicine, these courses must be satisfactorily completed.

The second course of study is to enter first a master's and then a doctoral course of study. These doctoral programs are 1-2 years and, similar to the master's-to-PhD route in conventional education, provide additional expertise and training in a more limited scope but deeper exploration of the area of study. For example, there are doctoral programs that focus on women's health and fertility, on research, and on oncology. Many of these programs require a thesis and/or thesis defense.

A third route of study is a direct admission doctoral program where the person begins after 90 hours of undergraduate credits to work toward their doctoral degree without "stopping" at a master's degree. These programs are a little shorter overall—typically five years—and allow the student to obtain the doctoral title more efficiently.

In all of the programs there is coursework in a classroom type of setting and clinical work where the students are learning patient interaction skills, physical exam skills, and technical skills related to acupuncture and ancillary techniques under supervision of an instructor. The level of responsibility and autonomy the student obtains increases over their years of study, similar to other medical educational structures for doctors and nurses, such that they are deemed competent to practice autonomously by the end of their training.

The training of acupuncturists and the certification of acupuncture schools is overseen by an accrediting body, the Accreditation Commission for Acupuncture and Herbal Medicine (ACAHM), which was founded in 1982 as the Accreditation Commission for Acupuncture and Oriental Medicine (ACAOM) and renamed to ACAHM in 2021. This body creates the structure of the number of hours in each type of coursework that must be present in the curriculum of a school, verifies that the coursework is sufficient to satisfy training requirements, and oversees the evolution of acupuncture education in the United States. The ACAHM itself is recognized by the U.S. Department of Education (USDE) and the Council for Higher Education Accreditation (CHEA).

---

### SEE ALSO

- "What other kinds of practitioners can use acupuncture needles?" *pg 149*
- "Do acupuncturists take board exams?" *pg 139*
- "References" *pg 181*

---

## Q. Do acupuncturists take board exams?

Like most medical practitioners, most acupuncturists do take board exams. Board examination is separate from licensing, but for most types of medical providers, board examinations are required for licensing. As an example, medical and osteopathic doctors must pass Step 1, Step 2, and Step 3 of the United States Medical Licensing Examination (USMLE) in order to become licensed as medical doctors (MD's) or doctors of osteopathic medicine (DO's) in the state(s) where they wish to practice.

In the United States, the body that administers the national board examinations is the National Certification Commission for Acupuncture and Oriental Medicine (NCCAOM). This board works closely with the Accreditation Commission for Acupuncture and Herbal Medicine (ACAHM) to ensure that the curriculum and the board examination match and that acupuncturists are safely and effectively trained following graduation and board examination.

The NCCAOM board examination is divided into four parts. To be board certified as "Diplomat of Acupuncture," the practitioner must take three of those four parts: Biomedicine, Foundations of Oriental Medicine, and Acupuncture. These persons designate their board certification by "Dipl Ac NCCAOM" behind their name.

To be board certified as a "Diplomat of Chinese Herbology," the practitioner must take three of those four NCCAOM examinations: Biomedicine, Foundations of Oriental Medicine, and Chinese Herbology.

To be board certified as a "Diplomat of Oriental Medicine," the practitioner must pass all four parts of the examination: Biomedicine, Foundations of Oriental Medicine, Acupuncture, and Chinese Herbology.

Most states require successful passage of some, if not all, NCCAOM board examinations before a practitioner is eligible for licensure in that state. As the scope of practice varies from state to state (as it does for all types of medical providers), it is up to the individual practitioner to undertake a course of study that will make them eligible for the necessary NCCAOM exams that will make them eligible for state licensure in the state(s) where they have chosen to practice.

California is the only state that has a separate board examination: the California Acupuncture Licensing Examination (CALE). The CALE is required to obtain licensure in California. Some California practitioners also chose to take NCCAOM exams—particularly if they think they might not always practice in California—but it is not required to do so for licensure.

In states where acupuncturists are not licensed medical providers, there are no requirements for board examinations. At the time of this writing, acupuncturists are not licensed in the states of Alabama, South Dakota, and Oklahoma

## SEE ALSO

- "Are acupuncturists licensed medical providers?" *pg 141*
- "How are acupuncturists trained?" *pg 137*
- "What other kinds of practitioners can use acupuncture needles?" *pg 149*
- "References" *pg 181*

## Q. Are acupuncturists licensed medical providers?

In most states in the US, yes, acupuncturists are licensed medical providers/practitioners. In Alabama, Oklahoma, and South Dakota, they are not yet licensed.

When a state requires licensure by creating a practice act, it also defines the scope of practice—what a practitioner is and is not allowed to do under their licensure. The scope of practice varies from state to state.

States requiring licensure also set up an oversight board so any complaints or concerns about a practitioner can be evaluated by an independent body that is outside of the practitioner-patient relationship.

The practitioner must obtain continuing education credits to continue to be licensed. Just like all healthcare providers, this is done so that each practitioner continues to learn and evolve as a clinician.

In states where there is no practice act and no licensure, these protections for the public are not in place.

An acupuncturist uses the letters "LAc" after their name to designate their status as a licensed acupuncturist. This is similar to designations such as "PhD," "MD," or "DO" that indicate various levels of professional training.

If you live in a state where there is no practice act or license for acupuncturists, you can still find a safe acupuncturist by looking for someone who has attended an accredited school, obtained a degree, and passed their NCCAOM exams, which you can verify by looking up their name on the NCCAOM website.

## SEE ALSO

- "Do acupuncturists take board exams?" *pg 139*
- "How are acupuncturists trained?" *pg 137*
- "What other kinds of practitioners can use acupuncture needles?" *pg 149*
- "References" *pg 181*

## Q. Where can I find a trusted, good, and/or safe acupuncturist?

Looking for someone who has a degree and a board certification (see above sections) is a good first step in finding a trusted, safe acupuncturist.

As has been outlined above, a degree and board certification ensures that the practitioner has gone through rigorous training, been supervised by experienced practitioners until they are deemed capable of functioning independently, and passed a series of challenging examinations created by a nationally-agreed upon standards of knowledge. This is the same model by which many other medical providers (medical doctors, nurses, therapists, etc.) are trained.

As a second step, you might ask other clinicians in similar fields who they recommend. Word gets around in communities. If everyone who needs a knee replacement is going to the same orthopedic surgeon and getting good results, it's a good bet that the person might be a good choice for your knee replacement surgery. If you ask the primary care providers in that community, they will know of that knee surgeon's reputation and pass along their name. Similarly, asking your healthcare team for an acupuncturist or two will clue you in to who has a good reputation in the community.

If clinicians in your area don't have a recommendation, asking friends and colleagues is another avenue. However, I would take these recommendations with a grain of salt. Most people place a disproportionate weight on the bedside manner of their practitioners—whether or not the person is "nice"—over technical skill. If you are mostly interested in bedside manner, asking for someone who is kind and gentle is perfect. If you are more interested in technique, results, and efficiency, then ask your friends for that. It's not outside the realm of possibility to think that you can find someone who is both kind and technically excellent, but just be aware of this potential bias when you receive the recommendations.

I would caution you similarly when looking at recommendations that people have put online. People who are angry and want to vent often do it online. People who are satisfied and delighted don't often take the time to write reviews. So be careful about judging a practitioner by their online "reputation" alone.

Know that you can always change practitioners. Just like changing your doctor or your massage therapist, going to see an acupuncturist for the first time is a kind of interview. Do you "click" with that person? Do you feel safe? Do you feel cared for? Did the treatment address your concerns, even in a small way? If you aren't feeling or thinking that this is the practitioner for you, it's completely normal to decide to go somewhere else.

I think about two people "clicking" in the following way. I'm chamomile tea. Some people are going to love chamomile tea and sing its praises. Some people are going to prefer rooibos or earl grey or green tea over chamomile. I can't change my chamomile'ness. I can be the best chamomile tea possible, but some people are just gonna prefer someone else. The people who don't like chamomile will find another practitioner that they click with. All of that is totally OK. Don't feel badly or have guilt if you are just not clicking with your practitioner. Find someone who is your cup of tea (couldn't resist—ha, ha).

Finally, the NCCAOM Professional Ethics and Disciplinary Committee has just released a new website that captures and publishes state and national information on all disciplinary matters involving licensed acupuncturists in the US. This site is called the Acupuncture National Discipline Database and allows a person to search for any practitioner's name. This database is unique because a practitioner cannot have an issue in one state and then apply for license in another state, hiding their misbehavior with a new application. This might sound shocking, but unfortunately the licensing system is not connected for any type of medical professional at the national level—it is all state-run and state-organized. The acupuncture profession is leading the way in ethical behavior by linking state-by-state data together in this way to protect the public.

---

**SEE ALSO**

- "Are acupuncturists licensed medical providers?" *pg 141*
- "Does acupuncture cause infections?" *pg 123*
- "Do acupuncturists take board exams?" *pg 139*
- "References" *pg 181*

---

## Q. What other kinds of things can an acupuncturist do?

While "acupuncture" technically refers to the use of the acupuncture needles in acupoints, being an acupuncturist is much more than just the placement of acupuncture needles. But answering the question of what else an acupuncturist might do is challenging because not all of the things below are within the scope of practice for acupuncturists in each state and not all techniques are used by all acupuncturists, even if it is within the scope of their practice. I'm going to discuss the most common techniques used by an acupuncturist. Please speak with your provider if you have questions regarding the kinds of things that they might be able to use in your particular treatment.

Cupping involves using suction cups placed at varying intensities on parts of the body. Cups might be made of glass or plastic and come in various sizes. An acupuncturist might use a technique in which they puncture the skin and draw out a small amount of blood with the cups in a technique called "bleeding cupping." When I have spastic muscles, this is one of my favorite treatment forms to receive. I'm not the only one—cupping is found in many culturally based forms of medicine.

Gua sha is a skin scraping technique. It is similar to Graston technique, which is used by many chiropractors and other body workers. "Gua" refers to the technique and "sha" refers to the reddish marks that the technique leaves behind. The sha generally fades over a few days, similar to the timeline of a bruise, but without going through all the color phases of a bruise. It generally doesn't turn green and brown but rather fades from pink/red/purple back to the person's skin color. I love this technique for tight tendons and for cold/flu symptoms.

Moxibustion is the use of an herb (*Artemisia vulgaris* or moxa) that is slowly smoldered directly on the skin or indirectly near the skin to transfer heat and healing oils into the body. Moxa is good for...well, all the things. Many practitioners can't use it—or don't like to use it—because of the smoke it generates. While there is "smokeless" moxa on the market, the moxa is very different texturally and heats up much hotter than regular moxa. I use smokeless moxa when I have to, but I prefer the regular stuff.

Acupuncturists also use techniques that are more 21st century. Lasers can be used to transfer infrared or other light waves into tissues or body parts to affect healing, similar to moxa but without the smoke and possible complaints from office building neighbors. E-stim might be used to connect needles in acupoints with a gentle electrical current that feels like a soft tap around the acupuncture needle.

The acupuncturist might use specialized massage or manipulation techniques like tui na or qi gong as a part of the treatment. Tui na feels much like a specialized massage and it is taught as such in acupuncture training programs. Qi Gong is a type of mind-body medicine that can be done on one's self or can be done by a practitioner on a patient.

An acupuncturist might also practice herbal medicine. This involves diagnosing the imbalances within your system and prescribing an herbal prescription, generally comprised of a group of herbs together called a "formula." The herbal medicines selected for the formula and their ratios are determined by the practitioner based on how the individual herbs function and how they function together. Herbs can be taken in a variety of ways such as a tea, powder, pill, capsule, or tincture. This kind of advice is based on thousands of years of clinical observation rather than randomized control trials. It is also based on using the whole herb or part of the herb: the leaf, the berry, the root, etc. It is not—like we do in biomedicine—taking a single chemical and putting it into a pill form. Acupuncturists sometimes learn about and use herbal medicines and/or nutraceuticals from other whole body systems of medicine such as Ayurveda or functional medicine.

Acupuncturists also typically use food prescriptions and dietary advice in their practice. This is generally far more specific than "you should eat more fruits and vegetables" and more like "you should eat less cantaloupe and more bitter melon." TEAM dietary advice is also attentive to circadian rhythms and times of the year. It will incorporate information about appropriate dietary modifications for the winter versus the summer, ideal times of day to eat particular foods, and how to cook or season food for that time of the year.

TEAM dietary recommendations are based on the foundational knowledge of traditional East Asian medicine as a whole-person construct and do not translate exactly into a biomedical paradigm.

For example, in conventional medicine, I would not recommend the one drug to a person who has dry eyes and is also having very heavy menstrual periods. Those are two separate concerns in bio-medicine and would be treated with eye drops and oral contra-ceptive pills. But goji berries (a food and an herb) are wonderful for treating both of those things simultaneously from a TEAM perspective, and I regularly recommend goji berries for the many women in my practice who have both dry eyes and heavy bleeding.

The line between herbal medicine and dietary advice is closely aligned, as I have tried to illustrate with the example above. Goji berries are a food. They are also an herb, *goji zi*, and used as such in herbal formulations. Not all herbs are foods. Not all foods are herbs. But there is some overlap.

Acupuncturists may also have some knowledge or expertise in Feng Shui and the use of color, sounds, and smells in health and healing contexts such as wearing earthy brown tones to ground yourself if you are feeling anxious or wearing red or orange if you need to boost your energy.

The list, then, of the most common techniques that an acupunc-turist can or might use in treating you is long and diverse. It's not just about needles. There are lots of other options with someone trained in TEAM!

## SEE ALSO

- "What is Traditional East Asian Medicine (TEAM)?" *pg 13*
- "References" *pg 181*

## Q. What other kinds of practitioners can use acupuncture needles?

Other types of medical providers are eligible to practice acupuncture and acupuncture-related techniques to varying extents. This is based on the state-specific practice act that defines the scope of practice of their primary licensure. I will go through only the more common, non-LAc types of practitioners who tend to use acupuncture here. For more information, please consult your state's department of professional regulation.

In addition to what is described below, all of the practitioners listed can take continuing education classes and courses to further their knowledge and understanding of acupuncture and acupuncture-related techniques.

### Nurses

In a few states, nurses can practice acupuncture but are required to have additional training. For most types of nurses, this means attending acupuncture school and becoming a licensed acupuncturist. Because of their biomedical education, some nurses may get credit for some or all of the biomedical coursework in the acupuncture curriculum. They would still need to take the NCCAOM Biomedicine examination and other examinations for board certification.

### Naturopathic doctors

Naturopathic doctors (ND's) are kinda like the primary care providers of the integrative medicine world. They know a great deal about a lot of different ways of treating the body with lifestyle, dietary changes, supplements and nutraceuticals, and body-based techniques. Their knowledge in these areas is both deep and wide. Most ND's receive training in TEAM as a part of their naturopathic schooling and—depending on their state's scope of practice—may or may not use acupuncture in their practice. Like acupuncturists, ND's are not licensed everywhere in the US and sometimes have to work with or for a chiropractor, medical doctor, or osteopathic doctor.

## Medical doctors and osteopathic doctors

In some states, medical doctors and doctors of osteopathic medicine (MD's and DO's) can practice acupuncture with or without additional training. Medical and osteopathic physicians also have avenues for advanced training and board certifications they can take under their licensure. For example, they can take 300+ hours of acupuncture-specific training and sit for a board exam administered by the American Board of Medical Acupuncture. When they do this, they achieve a DABMA or FABMA (designated as a "diplomat" at first, and then "fellow" after several years of good standing) acronym after their name.

## Chiropractors

Chiropractors (DC's) can practice acupuncture techniques with or without additional training, depending on their state's scope of practice. They can take a written and oral board exam administered by the American Board of Chiropractic Acupuncture (ABCA) after 300+ hours of training, which includes extensive hands-on components, clean needle techniques, moxibustion, and electrical stimulation techniques, to achieve the Diplomat of the American Board of Chiropractic Acupuncture (DABCA) acronym after their name. The Council of Chiropractic Acupuncture (CCA) supports and informs the ABCA by standardizing acupuncture training for chiropractic physicians.

### Physical therapists

More and more physical therapists (PT's) are using a restricted form of acupuncture called "dry needling." It is not legal in all states, and the training required varies widely between states. There is no national standard accrediting body or board examination for this form of acupuncture training for PT's. Dry needling is the only type of therapy that PT's are permitted to do that pierces the skin and penetrates into the tissues of the body.

## SEE ALSO

- "Does acupuncture interfere with my other medical treatments?" *pg 119*
- "Is acupuncture safe? What are the risks of acupuncture?" *pg 111*
- "What is the difference between acupuncture and dry needling?" *pg 151*
- "References" *pg 181*

## Q. What is the difference between acupuncture and dry needling?

Dry needling is commonly described as "acupuncture based on medical principles" rather than on TEAM theory, implying that TEAM theory is not medically sound and has no scientific basis. I find this definition exasperating, but let's spend some time talking about the differences. I am admittedly biased about this in the hands of some kinds of practitioners, but I will do my best to be as fair as possible.

## History of dry needling

Dry needling comes from work done by Dr. Janet Travell, a medical doctor who plotted a series of trigger points and then used needles to release the spastic muscles at those trigger points (As I have explained, trigger points are the same principle as "Ah shi" points). Trigger points were touted as a "new" discovery when she first wrote about them in 1942—an example of conventional medicine catching up with ancient medicine and giving it a new name instead of acknowledging TEAM's historical, medical, and cultural validity. Trigger points were injected with various medications by medical and osteopathic doctors to try to decrease the pain at the points.

Trigger point injections evolved into "wet needling," using the cutting tip of a phlebotomy needle to go beneath the skin and slice up knots or trigger points in muscles and connective tissue. The "wet" adjective referred to the amount of bleeding and bruising it caused. I have likened this to the equivalent of making *"ropa vieja"* out of the muscles under your skin with a phlebotomy needle. This creates a lot of tissue injury and a lot of pain.

The term "dry needling" was first described by Dr. Travell in 1983 in her book "Myofascial Pain and Dysfunction: Trigger Point Manual." Dry needling uses solid, filiform needles (ehem, acupuncture needles) because they are less painful and cause less bleeding.

Physical therapists (PT's) and other practitioners have adopted dry needling as a technique they use in the treatment of musculoskeletal pain and dysfunction. This is totally understandable because acupuncture ("Ah shi" points included) is very effective for treating pain. However, there is a lot of controversy around PT's doing dry needling.

## Scope of practice

The first is the issue of scope of practice. Licensed acupuncturists have extensive education on the use of needles, performing clean needle technique, and the supervised methods of needle placement. They are the acupuncture experts.

Medical and osteopathic doctors, chiropractors, naturopaths, and others are trained to perform techniques that penetrate the skin as a part of their "regular" education. These kinds of practitioners are commonly able to practice acupuncture under their medical, osteopathic, chiropractic or naturopathic license. This makes a certain degree of sense. If the practitioner can place a central line into a person's chest using the sensation of the tip of the needle to guide them, it is not a large logical leap to think that that same practitioner can feel the tissues using the tip of a small acupuncture needle. The scope of practice for these clinicians and the training that it takes to achieve licensure in their "regular" clinical jobs makes acupuncture, with appropriate acupuncture-specific training, a reasonable part of their practice.

Physical therapists are not taught to perform techniques that penetrate the skin in their regular training. Yet, a PT can take a weekend course and advertise that they are performing dry needling or acupuncture. This is like someone taking a weekend bread making class and calling themselves a pastry chef on a job application. It's just not the same level of knowledge and expertise.

Consequently, it is very confusing to patients who are looking to receive relief from pain by allowing themselves to be punctured by practitioners with very different training but the same kinds of needles. The reason that we define scope of practice for providers is so that patients can be kept safe.

## Patient safety

Dry needling is the only technique that PT's are allowed to use that penetrates the skin. Because they don't penetrate the skin as a part of their typical scope of practice, they don't have very much practice in learning to feel the different tissue layers with an instrument-like tip of the needle. They do have extensive training in feeling the tissues with their hands, but as a former surgeon, I can say that the sensation of a tumor under your hands through the skin is different from the feeling of a tumor at the end of a surgical instrument. Placing a large catheter into a blood vessel deep in the chest is different from feeling an artery right under the surface of the skin to place an arterial line. You have to learn to feel both. If you are not practiced in feeling both, you can miss subtle differences in the sensations of the tissues you feel through the needle handle and very easily get into areas where you should not force the needle.

Because PT's do not generally have extensive training requirements in feeling tissues this way, they are understandably more likely to go into non-muscle tissues like nerves, organs, and larger blood vessels. This is reflected in the higher number of adverse events reported with dry needling done by PT's than with acupuncture done by licensed acupuncturists, medical and osteopathic doctors, and chiropractors (all of whom have training in other forms of therapies that go beneath the skin). Because of inconsistent standards for reporting adverse events caused by dry needling, it is difficult to know whether or not the reported incidence is high, low, or accurate.

## Amount of acupuncture-specific training

Differences in state licensing requirements determine how much training a PT needs to do in order to use this technique and vary widely. PT's in some states (NY, CA, HI, OR, and WA at the time of this writing) are prohibited from performing the technique because of the classification of dry needling as a form of acupuncture. In some states, PT's can take a weekend class and begin to perform the technique. In other states, they must take longer training programs (300+ hours) before practicing on patients. To my knowledge, PT's are not licensed to perform trigger point injections as of the time of this writing.

## Summary

This is NOT meant to imply that PT's are in any way collectively "bad" people or untrustworthy practitioners. I have seen PT's for various health issues at several points in my life and have deep respect for the work that they do. I have friends that are PT's, have shared clinic space with PT's, and have collaborated with many PT's in the care of patients.

I am also not intending to imply that PT's are hiding the truth about adverse events that happen when they perform acupuncture techniques like dry needling. I believe that they are fundamentally good, honest, trustworthy, valuable, medical colleagues.

I can completely understand why PT's want to use dry needling as a part of their options for therapy. Like all medical providers, PT's as a group are motivated to help and care for their patients.

Acupuncture works very well for pain and musculoskeletal dysfunction, and those are the main reasons patients come to see them. Of course they want to use acupuncture because they want to help their patients in any way that they can.

However, I do not agree with the attempts to make it sound like dry needling is anything other than a form of acupuncture. It is using thin, solid needles to penetrate beneath the skin and affect changes in the tissues. That is acupuncture.

I also do not agree with the inference and assertions that TEAM and acupuncture are not based in sound, medical, scientific thinking. This is factually incorrect and culturally biased.

And finally I do not agree with the lack of training for PT's in this technique, which is leading to increased risk for patients and gives acupuncture a bad name by confusing patients and less-informed practitioners.

I think it is important for the public to know about this difference in primary training and acupuncture-specific training requirements so that people can make informed decisions about all the options available to them and the risks or benefits in the choices they have.

## SEE ALSO

- "Where do the needles go?" *pg 133*
- "Do the needles hurt?" *pg 114*
- "Can I use acupuncture with other methods for my issues?" *pg 98*
- "What other kinds of practitioners can use acupuncture needles?" *pg 149*

- "Does acupuncture interfere with my other medical treatments?" *pg 119*
- "References" *pg 181*

# CHAPTER EIGHT

# WHAT IS THE HISTORICAL BACKGROUND OF ACUPUNCTURE?

## Q. What is the history of acupuncture in the West?

There are many other books in which a person can find a comprehensive guide to TEAM history. My goal with this book is to give you the broad strokes version.

### Early history

One of the oldest forms of a recorded system of medicine is Ayurveda, which is about 5,000 years old. It is based on the ideas that natural phenomena such as earth, water, and air are related to human health and disease. Similar to the characteristics of the natural substances, humans exhibit stereotypes of physical form called doshas (vata, pitta, and kapha). For example, someone with a lot of earth in their doshas will tend to have a lot of inertia and dislike change, be a little heavier around the middle (spherical body shape), and be a person that others naturally gravitate to. The different doshas have tendencies to form various pathologies, need different kinds of foods and activity to stay healthy, and vary over a person's life depending on internal and external influences.

Each person has specific tendencies towards different doshas and the way to maintain health is to keep the doshas in balance with food, movement, herbal medicine, mindfulness and other lifestyle choices.

Traditional East Asian medicine (TEAM) is about 2,500 years old. It stems from Ayurveda and is similar in concept: natural phenomena are related to and influence health and patterns of disease. Health is defined as being in balance for your particular type. Disease and pathology arises when one part of the system overrides another or fails to support another.

The *Huang Di Nei Jing* (Yellow Emperor's Classic of Internal Medicine) is the oldest record of TEAM theory from 150 BCE. Many other theories have been brought forth over the years and incorporated into the medicine as it is currently practiced.

## *1700-1900*

When traders from the East India trading company went to China, they discovered that they could see farther out on the horizon when they got acupuncture on their earlobe—the reflection site for the eye in the auricular acupuncture microsystem. In order to make those effects last longer, they began piercing their earlobes at that site. The stereotype of a pirate with rings in their earlobes comes from acupuncture, and the earlobe is still the most common place where we pierce our ears today.

In the 1820s, books began to appear in French about acupuncture, and a physician named Franklin Bache published a report about using acupuncture to treat prison inmates for rheumatism and neuralgia. This led him to conclude that acupuncture's primary use was for mitigating and resolving pain—a presumption that still permeates people's conception of acupuncture to this day.

A German doctor, Philipp von Siebold, studied acupuncture and moxibustion in Japan and wrote several books on the subject in the 1830s-1850s. He reasoned that since the solid needles used by acupuncturists caused such an impressive reaction without drugs, the effect might be much stronger if one injected a drug directly into the person using a hollow needle. The concept of the hypodermic needle thus was born out of acupuncture and remains one of the most commonly used tools in conventional medicine.

In the late 1800's and early 1900's, acupuncture was used in the Civil War by surgeons and described in various field manuals, including Sir William Osler's *The Principles and Practice of Medicine*. A French diplomat to China, George Soulie de Morant, began to study acupuncture and wrote several books on the subject, which were translated into other languages and furthered western understanding of acupuncture.

## *1900-Present*

In the 1960s and 1970s, acupuncture was well established as a good treatment for pain and began to be considered as a potential alternative to anesthesia. It was used in place of anesthesia for hysterectomies, skin grafts, and other painful, invasive procedures. However, for a variety of reasons, it was difficult to reproduce the same results between patients. Neuroscientists like Ji-Sheng Han became curious about how exactly acupuncture impacts the central nervous system, contributing to our current understanding of how the opioid, enkephalin, and beta-endorphin chemical messengers influence the brain and nervous system.

Around the same time, the Nixon administration was allowed to visit previously-closed communist China for the first time. Traveling with Nixon's press core was one of the editors of the New York Times, James Reston. He had to have an emergency appendectomy while in China and described the use of acupuncture in treating his post-operative pain in an article on the front page of the NYT. Several doctors from the US, including Nixon's personal physician, went to China and corroborated accounts of acupuncture being used for surgical analgesia.

In the 1980's, interest in acupuncture continued to build. The National Institutes of Health (NIH) and World Health Organization (WHO) standardized nomenclature, scope of practice, and training standards. Medical, chiropractic, and osteopathic doctors began to learn acupuncture, and licensed acupuncturists were defined as clinicians.

In 1997, the NIH acknowledged acupuncture's use for pain relief, stroke rehabilitation, nausea after surgery or chemotherapy, headaches, asthma, and other ailments. In the same study, the NIH recommended that acupuncture be taught in all medical schools.

National Health Interview Surveys demonstrated that between 2002 and 2007, acupuncture use by adults increased by 1 million people and an estimated 3.1 million U.S. adults and 150,000 children had used acupuncture in 2006. The data from the latest NHIS in 2022 is just beginning to be published at the time of this writing, but it indicates that acupuncture use again has gone up since the last survey.

The U.S. Bureau of Labor Statistics has recently established "acupuncturist" as an official occupation (29-1291) and now tracks employment and wages data for acupuncturists that are employed by another entity. Acupuncture and acupuncturists are being increasingly integrated into conventional medicine offices, colleges and professional schools, and hospitals. However, employment and wage data is problematic because most acupuncturists are self-employed and the US BLS tracking won't capture that information.

This is a very brief overview of the subject and its contributions to conventional medicine, but I hope I have spurred your curiosity on the subject. There are several historically-oriented references in that section of this book. [3]

---

### SEE ALSO

- "What is Traditional East Asian Medicine (TEAM)?" *pg 13*
- "How does the thought theory of acupuncture differ from conventional medicine?" *pg 163*
- "References" *pg 181*

---

## Q. How does the thought theory of acupuncture differ from conventional medicine?

TEAM is conceptualized in a similar way to conventional medicine. Physical problems are addressed by fixing the physical mechanism. Internal problems are addressed by taking substances internally. In conventional medicine, this plays out as surgery and physical therapy for mechanical issues and as pharmaceuticals, supplements, and lifestyle for internal medical issues. Hence the broad designation of "surgical problems" and "medical problems,"

---

3   Because of the focus of the lineage from Ayurveda to traditional Chinese medicine to TEAM to the west, this history does not include other traditional or indigenous systems of medicine such as Native American medicine or Aboriginal medicine and their potential impacts on current acupuncture understanding and practice today.

and doctors broadly being classified as either surgeons or medical doctors.

In TEAM, the parallels to surgery and physical therapy are acupuncture, tui na, cupping, moxibustion, gua sha and other mechanical things done to a person's physical, external body by a practitioner on a patient. The parallels to treatments for internal medical problems are herbal medicine, qi gong, and dietetics. In this way, the two forms of medicine are similar.

What is not similar is the approach of adding additional information to the accepted theories of thought. In conventional medicine, old theories are typically discarded in place of new ones. In TEAM, new theories don't necessarily replace the old ones: they may be used alongside one another.

In conventional medicine, for example, the idea of "spontaneous putrefaction" (tissues rotting spontaneously) was displaced by an understanding of bacteria, molds, fungi , and viruses as causes of disease. This slowly evolved through the notions of alcoholic fermentation, the importance of handwashing, Louis Pasteur's work (pasteurization), the discovery of penicillin, and the work of many more scientists and researchers. Once scientists had solid evidence that bacteria were causing disease, they didn't refer to it as a spontaneous event anymore and discarded the old theories in favor of the new germ theory.

The Yellow Emperor's Classic (*Huang Di Nei Jing*) contains the oldest records of TEAM theory. There are theories in which the Five Elements or Phases interact in particular ways. There are theories of "Cold Disease" (*Shang Han Lun*) and of "Heat Disease" (*Wen Beng Tiao Bian*). All of these theories (and many others) are still practiced and used by acupuncturists all over the world each day. They are not mutually exclusive to each other: they are all simultaneously true and effective. I use each of them in my treatment of patients regularly.

Similar to the application of the scientific method in conventional medicine, each TEAM theory was slowly conceptualized and put to rigorous examination, debate, and experimentation. The various theories evolved over time as each was treated with suspicion at first and gradually gained acceptance as its efficacy was confirmed. But the big difference between conventional medicine and TEAM is that new theories in TEAM were layered as alternatives to old—not as replacements like in conventional medicine.

Because it is too intricate to try to explain this in the context of TEAM in this book, I will use a perhaps more familiar parallel to illustrate my point. If you go to a talk therapist, you know that you are going to be expected to talk about yourself, your feelings, your relationships, and your stressors. But the framework (theory) of how you do that can be very different. If you see a therapist who focuses on Jungian psychology, you might be asked to talk about your feelings in the context of your dreams. If you see someone who specializes in Imago Relationship Therapy, they might ask you to talk about your feelings in the context of your family of origin and examine how those dynamics are playing out in your adult life. Cognitive Behavioral Therapists will emphasize changing your thought patterns when you find that they are not serving you. Which one is right?

The answer is that they all are simultaneously "true" and effective methods of talk therapy. Further, the correctness and efficacy of one does not negate the other. They are all pathways of healing. The reasons a person might pick one over another will vary widely, but I think it is fair to say that healing can take place with all of those modalities of talk therapy. If a therapist is trained in all of them, they can then tailor their approach to the needs of the client.

Similarly, when I am treating a patient, I am looking at the person through the lenses of all the TEAM theories that I know and trying to tailor my treatment to the needs of the individual in front of me. I default most naturally to Five Element theory, but that doesn't mean that I ignore other theories when I am looking at a person's needs for that session in that moment. I don't pick Five Element as "correct" and the others as "incorrect." They are all simultaneously true and useful to me, despite—or perhaps because of—their subtle disagreements in how the body is constructed.

I am not doing that in conventional medicine. I am not thinking at the same time about spontaneous putrefaction and germ theory and bacteria as a cause of disease when I am evaluating the imbalance of bacteria, yeasts, and viruses in someone's microbiome. I disregarded the old theories and replaced them with the new ones. This is Newtonian in its approach: that a new idea supplants the old one.

The idea of "multiple truths being simultaneously correct" is aligned with modern Einsteinian physics. TEAM is, in this sense, a quantum medicine in which multiple theories can be simultaneously present, effective, and true. As such, I'm not limited by Newtonian, black and white thinking when I approach a person I am seeing for acupuncture. I can use *Shang Han Lun* for you today, Five Element for you next week, and *Wen Bing* for you the week afterwards. Or I can use Five Element to pick your acupuncture points and *Wen Bing* to pick your herbal medicine. It all works. It's just a framework—the perspective of looking at a room through the door or the window. Same room, but different perspectives available to me within each of the possible theories.

You can see that this is a very different mindset between the two types of medicine, and is, in my opinion, one of the reasons that conventional practitioners and acupuncturists struggle to communicate with each other. One is looking at diagnosis from a right-wrong, decision tree kind of perspective. In the conventional paradigm, there is one correct diagnosis and one ideal treatment for a given problem. TEAM looks at diagnosis from the perspective that all body parts are interconnected and influencing each other at the same time, hence there can be more than one appropriate diagnosis and the diagnoses can be addressed in many different ways.

I appreciate that TEAM makes me think about the assumptions I made in medical school when I was training to be a doctor. I thought I understood how the body worked...or at least could figure it out if I read and studied enough. I now believe that living creatures are far more complex than we imagine, and, at least speaking for my little pea brain, I don't think I could possibly understand it all even if I had many lifetimes to figure it out.

Studying TEAM has also taught me that it's not always in the best interest of the patient to treat pathology as an isolated problem in an isolated organ or system. I am glad that conventional medicine is also moving in the direction of tailored treatment designed to address the spectacular complexity of the individual. As a medical doctor and licensed acupuncturist, I look forward to continuing to learn and grow in my appreciation for the wonder of human bodies and all that they can do...no matter what educational perspective I take. Medicine, in all its forms, is truly amazing.

## SEE ALSO

- "What is Traditional East Asian Medicine (TEAM)?" *pg 13*
- "How does an acupuncturist formulate a diagnosis and treatment plan?" *pg 56*
- "What does acupuncture actually do?" *pg 72*
- "Is acupuncture just placebo?" *pg 82*

# CHAPTER NINE

# HOW DO I PAY FOR ACUPUNCTURE TREATMENTS?

## Q. Do any insurance companies cover acupuncture?

The short answer is yes, some do. As to exactly what is covered, what diagnosis is necessary for coverage, the dollars reimbursed to the acupuncturist for services rendered, and other such specifics, it varies widely depending on the insurance company and the policy.

### How it works

You are likely aware that insurance companies have a wide variety of policies that offer various levels of coverage. The insurance company and the policy details describe the kinds of services that a person can receive under that plan. The kind of policy you have as a patient is a relationship between you (the patient) and the insurance company.

Just like medical doctors, therapists, and hospitals, acupuncturists can choose or not to be paneled by an insurance company. This means that the acupuncturist signs a contract with the insurance company to accept their rates of reimbursement. We then say that the acupuncturist "takes the insurance" policy for that particular company. In exchange, the acupuncturist is listed on the insurance company's website as a part of the list of clinicians the patient can see under their policy.

Without getting too heavily into the politics of insurance, the idea is that an insurance policy takes money from a patient (and/or employer) that goes into a large pool of funding that then is spent when a patient needs health services. The insurance company is a middle man, parsing out funds to clinicians on behalf of a patient for services rendered. The client of the insurance company (stockholders aside) is you, the patient.

The insurance company is not financially motivated to provide the clinician with any reimbursement, nor is it financially motivated to provide additional services not currently supplied...unless it can be shown that the services provided save the insurance company money.

Acupuncture is being covered by more insurance companies and found more often in insurance policies because it is exactly that kind of service. It is an effective, safe treatment for a wide variety of medical problems and is often much less expensive than a lifetime of medications or a surgical procedure.

Because *you* are their client and they are financially motivated to keep *you* happy and buying their policy, it is most effective for you to call them or write to them to ask them to cover acupuncture services. You also have the option to look for other insurance policies that cover acupuncture services.

---

**SEE ALSO**

- "How do I submit to my insurance company for reimbursement?" *pg 171*

---

## Q. How do I submit to my insurance company for reimbursement?

This question assumes that the acupuncturist doesn't "take" your insurance policy, so I am going to explain the procedure for how to apply for reimbursement from your insurance company directly.

### *Policy Coverage*

It is best to find out ahead of time (in writing if at all possible) what your policy covers. Ask specifically what diagnoses need to be used and what treatment codes need to be used in order to maximize reimbursement.

Prepare yourself that your insurance company may be a little reluctant to give you this information. They are not financially motivated to reimburse anyone because this cuts into their profits, and they are business people who are in business to make money for themselves and their shareholders. But as their customer, I suggest you insist on this information.

### *Superbill*

Insurance companies require two primary pieces of information for reimbursement: the diagnosis code (ICD-10 = International

Classification of Diseases, 10th version) and the treatment or procedure code (Current Procedural Terminology = CPT). Most acupuncturists can provide the ICD-10 and CPT codes for you on a sheet of paper called a "superbill" at the end of your treatment. Your acupuncturist is generally very willing to work with you so that they are using the codes that your insurance company has specified must be used for reimbursement. If, for example, I am seeing someone for headaches, digestive issues, dizziness and sleep problems but the insurance company will only reimburse for headaches, that is the diagnosis code that I will put on your superbill. I'm not lying or being in any way unethical. I am just telling the insurance company that I have treated you for one of the problems that is on their list of reasons why they will reimburse for acupuncture treatment.

In the same way, sometimes insurance companies will reimburse for evaluation and management (E&M) codes but not for acupuncture codes. Because I always spend a large proportion of my time talking to, examining, and making a plan for my patients, I feel very comfortable using E&M codes for most patients. For acupuncture providers who are not doctors, this can be a little more challenging because there are specific rules about how often you can bill an E&M code, how many minutes you are spending during the visit doing E&M vs other things, etc. But most acupuncturists will work with you to do their best to help you maximize your reimbursement.

## Submission

You have to check with your insurance company about the precise procedures for submission. Once they tell you how to submit, you send in a copy of the superbill, keeping one for your records. Most insurance companies have an online method of submission through a patient portal.

## *In or Out of Network*

As discussed previously, the acupuncturist you see may or may not be paneled with a particular insurance company. If they are "in network" or paneled, they can receive reimbursement directly from the insurance company, and you don't have to go through all of this because the acupuncturist will submit directly to the insurance company. If they are "out of network" or not paneled, the money they bill you for care might count toward your "out of network" deductible. This is why it is worthwhile to submit for reimbursement for acupuncture if you have any acupuncture coverage in your policy.

## *FSA and HSA Money*

You can also use a Flexible Spending Account (FSA) or Healthcare Savings Account (HSA) to cover your acupuncture treatments in most cases. FSA and HSA monies are taken out of a person's pay pretax. This money is held in an account to be spent on healthcare expenses over the course of the year.

### SEE ALSO

- "Do any insurance companies cover acupuncture?" *pg 169*

## Q. Does Medicare cover acupuncture?

Medicare covers 20 treatments of acupuncture for low back pain by a provider described in the Medicare Act. That is the only diagnostic code currently covered by Medicare.

While the Department of Health and Human Services can determine what Medicare does and does not cover, it cannot determine the kinds of providers that Medicare can reimburse for care. That takes an act of Congress.

Acupuncturists are not currently on the list of providers that can receive Medicare reimbursement, so the patients who would be eligible to receive services for low back pain must either go to a medical doctor, doctor of osteopathic medicine, or chiropractor for these services or must see an acupuncturist who is working under the "supervision" of a medical, osteopathic, or chiropractic clinician.

There is a bill currently (2023) in Congress that would add licensed acupuncturists to the list of practitioners that the U.S. Centers for Medicare and Medicaid Services (CMS) can reimburse for services rendered. If this is something that you would like to see done, please call your Congressperson and Senator and ask them to support the "Acupuncture for Our Seniors Act" (H.R. 3133) put forth by Rep. Judy Chu (D-CA) and Rep. Brian Fitzpatrick (R-PA).

## Q. Does Medicaid cover acupuncture?

Several clinical studies have been done on the efficacy and cost savings of providing acupuncture under Medicaid. As a consequence, in a few states, Medicaid covers acupuncture.

Please contact your state's Medicaid office to determine whether or not you have coverage in your state.

If your state does not cover acupuncture under Medicaid, look for a community acupuncture clinic, a school of acupuncture, or acupuncture within a larger healthcare clinic for affordable options for care.

## SEE ALSO

- "How much does a treatment cost?" *pg 175*
- "How can I find low cost options for acupuncture treatment?" *pg 176*

## Q. How much does a treatment cost?

As with the costs of all goods and services, the cost of acupuncture varies by geographic location and the expertise of the practitioner.

For a one-on-one treatment, the cost generally varies between $50 and $180, with the national average close to $85.

Community acupuncture clinics are typically on a sliding scale of $30-65 per treatment.

Most practitioners charge a little more for the initial intake and treatment and then have a set rate for follow-up visits going forward.

Please visit the websites of acupuncturists in your area for more specifics on their charges and options for treatment.

## Q. How can I find low cost options for acupuncture treatment?

There are several ways to save money on acupuncture treatment. One is to go to an acupuncture school for treatment. Similar to going to an academic medical school or clinic where a future doctor (medical student and/or resident) is being supervised by more senior, fully trained clinicians, training programs for acupuncture students involve supervision by fully trained acupuncturists. A student will evaluate a patient and then report their findings to a senior acupuncturist, who will evaluate the patient themselves and guide the treatment of the patient. Treatments in these kinds of settings are substantially lower than in private clinics. In some areas, they can be as low as $20.

Another way to keep costs low for acupuncture treatment is by going to a community acupuncture clinic. In this kind of setting, multiple patients are seen in a single large room. They are typically arranged in reclining chairs with music and/or ambient noise playing in the background. The acupuncturist treats each person in turn. The patient then relaxes with needles in place while the acupuncturist moves to the next person. Because the acupuncturist can see multiple patients per hour in this kind of setting, the cost tends to be lower and/or on a sliding scale of $30-65 (again depending on location and experience of the practitioner).

When I was working at a medical school and when I had a private practice with multiple acupuncturists working for me, I had an auricular acupuncture clinic. Using the ear as a microsystem still allows me to address the whole person extremely effectively. It is very quick because no one has to take their shoes off or get positioned on a table. I was seeing 20-30 people each hour in this kind of setting (with a helper) and charging $5-10 per treatment. I loved it because it was very inexpensive and effective for the patient and very quick and efficient for the practitioner. Finding these kinds of clinics is difficult because it is usually not the way the entire clinic is set up. For me, this was something that I did for a half day once a week. I would not have been able to stay in business at that price point, but I did love giving back to the community in this way.

Finally, some practitioners offer options for "herbal medicine only" kinds of treatments. These tend to be less expensive than getting acupuncture itself. Because herbal medicine can also be a very effective form of treatment, this can be another option if financially it is not possible to receive regular acupuncture.

DEMYSTIFYING ACUPUNCTURE

# CONCLUSION

I thank you for reading this book. I have enjoyed putting it together for you and giggled out loud more than once remembering all the conversations that I have had over the years leading up to this point. I hope that I have adequately introduced you to the idea of acupuncture and that, with this new knowledge, you might consider using traditional East Asian medicine to service some of your healthcare needs. It's really good stuff, this medicine. I don't want you to miss out.

# REFERENCES

Reference List for This Book

*Anticoagulant Medicine Safety:*

Mcculloch M, Nachat A, Schwartz J, Casella-Gordon V, Cook J. *Acupuncture safety in patients receiving anticoagulants: a systematic review.* Perm J. 2015 Winter;19(1):68-73. doi: 10.7812/ TPP/14-057. Epub 2014 Nov 24. PMID: 25432001; PMCID: PMC4315381.

Leem J. *Does acupuncture increase the risk of bleeding in patients taking warfarin?* Integr Med Res. 2015 Jun;4(2):119-121. doi: 10.1016/j.imr.2015.04.001. Epub 2015 Apr 22. PMID: 28664117; PMCID: PMC5481786.

*Acupuncture Meridians and TEAM Theory:*

Hua, Shou. *Shi Si Jing Fa Hui (Expression of the Fourteen Meridians)* at National Libraries of Medicine Digital Collections

https://www.nlm.nih.gov/exhibition/historicalanatomies/ huashou_home.html

**Chant B, Dieberg G, Madison J.** *Cross-cultural differences in acupuncture: A review.* Aust J Acupunct Chinese Med 2016; 10:12-8. https://hdl.handle.net/1959.11/19702.

**Deadman, Peter, et al.** *A Manual of Acupuncture.* Journal of Chinese Medicine, 1998. ISBN 0951054651

**Ikeda, Masakazu.** *The Practice of Japanese Acupuncture and Moxibustion: Classic Principles in Action.* Eastland Press, 2005. ISBN 0939616432

**Maciocia, Giovanni.** *The Foundations of Chinese Medicine: A Comprehensive Text.* Churchill Livingstone, 2015. ISBN 0702052167

**Young Kim, Angie.** *Decoding Korean Acupuncture: Korean Constitutional Acupuncture, Joseon Acupuncture, and Sa Arm Acupuncture.* Kindle, 2021. ISBN: 979-8790929939

*Dry Needling:*

**Boyce D, Wempe H, Campbell C, Fuehne S, Zylstra E, Smith G, Wingard C, Jones R.** *Adverse Events Associated with Therapeutic Dry Needling.* Int J Sports Phys Ther. 2020 Feb;15(1):103-113. PMID: 32089962; PMCID: PMC7015026.

**Kearns GA, Brismée JM, Riley SP, Wang-Price S, Denninger T, Vugrin M.** *Lack of standardization in dry needling dosage and adverse event documentation limits outcome and safety reports: a scoping review of randomized clinical trials.* J Man Manip Ther. 2023 Apr;31(2):72-83. doi: 10.1080/10669817.2022.2077516. Epub 2022 May 23. PMID: 35607259; PMCID: PMC10013441.

## History:

Han JS. A*cupuncture: neuropeptide release produced by electrical stimulation of different frequencies.* Trends Neurosci. 2003 Jan;26(1):17-22. doi: 10.1016/s0166-2236(02)00006-1. PMID: 12495858.

Jaiswal YS, Williams LL. *A glimpse of Ayurveda - The forgotten history and principles of Indian traditional medicine.* J Tradit Complement Med. 2016 Feb 28;7(1):50-53. doi: 10.1016/j. jtcme.2016.02.002. PMID: 28053888; PMCID: PMC5198827.

Lu, Dominic and Gabriel Lu. *An Historical Review and Perspective on the Impact of Acupuncture on U.S. Medicine and Society.* Medical Acupuncture Journal, Oct 2013

## Placebo:

Beecher HK. *The Powerful Placebo.* JAMA. 1955;159(17):1602-1606. doi:10.1001/jama.1955.02960340022006

Dobs, A. *A little better than placebo is still better than nothing.* Nat Med 19, 962 (2013). https://doi.org/10.1038/nm0813-962

Kaptchuk, Ted and Franklin Miller, PhD. *Placebo Effects in Medicine.* Perspectives NEJM. 2015. https://pubmed.ncbi.nlm. nih.gov/12110735/

http://programinplacebostudies.org/wp-content/ uploads/2015/07/PerspectivesNEJM-KaptchukMiller.pdf

Peters, David ed. *Understanding the Placebo Effect in Complementary Medicine: Theory, Practice and Research.* Churchill Livingstone Harcourt Publishers Limited, 2001.

Sihvonen R, Paavola M, Malmivaara A, Itälä A, Joukainen A, Nurmi H, Kalske J, Järvinen TL; Finnish Degenerative Meniscal Lesion Study (FIDELITY) Group. *Arthroscopic partial meniscectomy versus sham surgery for a degenerative meniscal tear.* N Engl J Med. 2013 Dec 26;369(26):2515-24. doi: 10.1056/ NEJMoa1305189. PMID: 24369076.

Sihvonen R, Paavola M, Malmivaara A, Itälä A, Joukainen A, Nurmi H, Kalske J, Ikonen A, Järvelä T, Järvinen TAH, Kanto K, Karhunen J, Knifsund J, Kröger H, Kääriäinen T, Lehtinen J, Nyrhinen J, Paloneva J, Päiväniemi O, Raivio M, Sahlman J, Sarvilinna R, Tukiainen S, Välimäki VV, Äärimaa V, Toivonen P, Järvinen TLN; FIDELITY (Finnish Degenerative Meniscal Lesion Study) Investigators. *Arthroscopic partial meniscectomy versus placebo surgery for a degenerative meniscus tear: a 2-year follow-up of the randomised controlled trial.* Ann Rheum Dis. 2018 Feb;77(2):188-195. doi: 10.1136/annrheumdis-2017-211172. Epub 2017 May 18. PMID: 28522452; PMCID: PMC5867417.

## Tongue and Pulse Diagnosis:

Bilton, Karen, Leon Hammer, and Chris Zaslawski. *Contemporary Chinese Pulse Diagnosis: A Modern Interpretation of an Ancient and Traditional Method.* J Acupunct Meridian Stud 2013;6(5):227e233

## Authors Writing From Cultural Authority

Chen Ping (editor in chief), *History and Development of Traditional Chinese Medicine.* IOS Press, 2000. ISBN 9051993242

Dai-zhao, Zhang. *Alleviating the Side Effects of Cancer Treatment.* People's Medical Publishing House, 2006. ISBN 7117087021

Feng, Youu-Lan, and Derk Bodde. *A Short History of Chinese Philosophy*. Free Press, 1997. ISBN 0684836343

Hur, Inn-hee. *Korean Medicine: A Holistic Way to Health and Healing*. Seoul Selection, 2013. ISBN 8997639390

Ikeda, Masakazu. *The Practice of Japanese Acupuncture and Moxibustion: Classic Principles in Action*. Eastland Press, 2005. ISBN 0939616432

Kuriyama, Shigehisa. *The Expressiveness of the Body and the Divergence of Greek and Chinese Medicine*. Princeton University Press, 2002. ISBN 0942299892

Li, Xiumin et al. *Traditional Chinese Medicine, Western Science, and the Fight Against Allergic Disease*. WSPC, 2016. ISBN 9814733695

Liu, Yanchi. *The Essential Book of Traditional Chinese Medicine, Vol. 1: Theory*. Columbia University Press, 1988. ISBN 0231103573

Liu, Yanchi. *The Essential Book of Traditional Chinese Medicine, Vol. 2: Clinical Practice*. Columbia University Press,1995. ISBN 023110359X

Matsumoto, Kiiko and Stephen Birch. *Five Elements and Ten Stems: Nan Ching Theory, Diagnostics and Practice*. Paradigm Publications, 1983. ISBN 0912111356

Ni, Maoshing PhD. *The Yellow Emperor's Classic of Medicine: A New Translation of the Neijing Suwen with Commentary*. Shambahala, 1995. ISBN 1570620806

Tzu, Lao. *Tao Te Ching (The Book of the Way)*. Many translations and editions to chose from.

Xinyi Gong, Zoey. *The Five Elements Cookbook: A Guide to Traditional Chinese Medicine with Recipes for Everyday Healing.* Harvest, 2023. ISBN 0358622190

Yan-heng, Wang. *Treatment of Depressive Disorders with Chinese Medicine: an Integrative Approach.* People's Medical Publishing House, 2010. ISBN 7117127295

Young Kim, Angie. *Decoding Korean Acupuncture: Korean Constitutional Acupuncture, Joseon Acupuncture, and Sa Arm Acupuncture.* Kindle, 2021. ISBN: 979-8790929939

## More Reading for Medical Professionals

### Medical Journal Articles:

Chiang, Poney. *What is the Point of Acupuncture? Medical Acupuncture.* Apr 2015.67-80.http://doi.org/10.1089/acu.2015.1093

Hao JJ, Mittelman M. *Acupuncture: past, present, and future.* Glob Adv Health Med. 2014 Jul;3(4):6-8. doi: 10.7453/gahmj.2014.042. PMID: 25105069; PMCID: PMC4104560.

Lee, Melissa, Ryan Longenecker, Samuel Lo, and Poney Chiang. *Distinct Neuroanatomical Structures of Acupoints Kidney 1 to Kidney 8: A Cadaveric Study.* Medical Acupuncture. Feb 2019.19-28.http://doi.org/10.1089/acu.2018.1325

Liu S, Wang Z, Su Y, Qi L, Yang W, Fu M, Jing X, Wang Y, Ma Q. *A neuroanatomical basis for electroacupuncture to drive the vagal-adrenal axis.* Nature 2021;598:641-5. 10.1038/s41586-021-04001-4.

Lu DP, Lu GP. *An Historical Review and Perspective on the Impact of Acupuncture on U.S. Medicine and Society.* Med Acupunct. 2013 Oct;25(5):311-316. doi: 10.1089/acu.2012.0921. PMID: 24761180; PMCID: PMC3796320.

Meltz, Leah, Daniel Ortiz, and Poney Chiang. *The Anatomical Relationship Between Acupoints of the Face and the Trigeminal Nerve.* Medical Acupuncture. Aug 2020.181-193.http://doi.org/10.1089/acu.2020.1413

Nahin RL, Rhee A, Stussman B. *Use of complementary health approaches overall and for pain management by US adults in 2002, 2012 and 2022.* JAMA. DOI:10.1001/jama.2023.26775 (2024)

Nguyen LT, Kaptchuk TJ, Davis RB, Nguyen G, Pham V, Tringale SM, Loh YL, Gardiner P. *The Use of Traditional Vietnamese Medicine Among Vietnamese Immigrants Attending an Urban Community Health Center in the United States.* J Altern Complement Med. 2016 Feb;22(2):145-53. doi: 10.1089/acm.2014.0209. Epub 2015 Dec 2. PMID: 26630121; PMCID: PMC4761825. doi: 10.1089/acm.2014.0209

Nielsen A, Dusek JA, Taylor-Swanson L, Tick H. *Acupuncture Therapy as an Evidence-Based Nonpharmacologic Strategy for Comprehensive Acute Pain Care: The Academic Consortium Pain Task Force White Paper Update.* Pain Med. 2022 Aug 31;23(9):1582-1612. doi: 10.1093/pm/pnac056. PMID: 35380733; PMCID: PMC9434305.

Sihvonen R, Paavola M, Malmivaara A, Itälä A, Joukainen A, Nurmi H, Kalske J, Järvinen TL; Finnish Degenerative Meniscal Lesion Study (FIDELITY) Group. *Arthroscopic partial meniscectomy versus sham surgery for a degenerative meniscal tear.* N Engl J Med. 2013 Dec 26;369(26):2515-24. doi: 10.1056/NEJMoa1305189. PMID: 24369076.

Sihvonen R, Paavola M, Malmivaara A, Itälä A, Joukainen A, Nurmi H, Kalske J, Ikonen A, Järvelä T, Järvinen TAH, Kanto K, Karhunen J, Knifsund J, Kröger H, Kääriäinen T, Lehtinen J, Nyrhinen J, Paloneva J, Päiväniemi O, Raivio M, Sahlman J, Sarvilinna R, Tukiainen S, Välimäki VV, Äärimaa V, Toivonen P, Järvinen TLN; FIDELITY (Finnish Degenerative Meniscal Lesion Study) Investigators. *Arthroscopic partial meniscectomy versus placebo surgery for a degenerative meniscus tear: a 2-year follow-up of the randomised controlled trial.* Ann Rheum Dis. 2018 Feb;77(2):188-195. doi: 10.1136/annrheumdis-2017-211172. Epub 2017 May 18. PMID: 28522452; PMCID: PMC5867417.

Vickers AJ, Cronin AM, Maschino AC, et al. *Acupuncture for Chronic Pain: Individual Patient Data Meta-analysis.* Arch Intern Med. 2012;172(19):1444-1453. doi:10.1001/archinternmed.2012.3654

### References From Medical Websites:

*NIH/NCCIH Description of Acupuncture*
https://www.nccih.nih.gov/health/acupuncture-what-you-need-to-know

*Center for Medicare and Medicaid Services (CMS) Coverage of Acupuncture for Low Back Pain*
https://www.cms.gov/medicare-coverage-database/view/nca-cal-decision-memo.aspx?proposed=N&NCAId=295

https://www.medicare.gov/coverage/acupuncture

*Acupuncture Within the VA Whole Health System*
https://www.va.gov/WHOLEHEALTH/professional-resources/
Acupuncture.asp

*International Association for the Study of Pain (IASP) Fact Sheet on Acupuncture for Pain Relief*
https://www.iasp-pain.org/resources/fact-sheets/
acupuncture-for-pain-relief/

# More Reading for the General Public

## *Books:*

Bleeker, Deborah. *Acupuncture Points Handbook: A Patient's Guide to the Locations and Functions of over 400 Acupuncture Points.* Draycott Publishing, 2017. ISBN 1940146208.

Beinfield, Harriet and Efrem Korngold. *Between Heaven and Earth: A Guide to Chinese Medicine.* Ballantine Books, 1992. ISBN 0345379748

Hammer, Leon. *Dragon Rises, Red Bird Flies: Psychology and Chinese Medicine.* Eastland Press, 2005. ISBN 0939616475

Kaptchuk, Ted J. *The Web That Has No Weaver: Understanding Chinese Cedicine.* Congdon & Weed, 1983. ISBN 0865530211

Pitchford, Paul. *Healing with Whole Foods.* North Atlantic Books, 2002. ISBN 9781556434303

Reichstein, Gail. *Wood Becomes Water: Chinese Medicine in Everyday Life.* Kodansha USA, 1998. ISBN 1568365888

## *Web resources:*

*Acupuncture Within the VA Whole Health System*

https://www.va.gov/WHOLEHEALTH/professional-resources/
Acupuncture.asp

*Breast Cancer.org Description of Acupuncture*

https://www.breastcancer.org/treatment/complementary-therapy/
types/acupuncture

*Center for Medicare and Medicaid Services (CMS) Coverage of
Acupuncture for Low Back Pain*

https://www.cms.gov/medicare-coverage-database/view/nca-
cal-decision-memo.aspx?proposed=N&NCAId=295

https://www.medicare.gov/coverage/acupuncture

*Cleveland Clinic Article "Acupuncture Myths Debunked"*

https://health.clevelandclinic.org/
acupuncture-10-biggest-myths-and-facts-2/

*Cleveland Clinic Description of Acupuncture*

https://my.clevelandclinic.org/health/
treatments/4767-acupuncture

*Healthline article on Acupuncture*

https://www.healthline.com/health/
acupuncture-how-does-it-work-scientifically

*International Association for the Study of Pain (IASP) Fact Sheet on Acupuncture for Pain Relief*
https://www.iasp-pain.org/resources/fact-sheets/acupuncture-for-pain-relief/

*Johns Hopkins Medicine Article on Acupuncture*
https://www.hopkinsmedicine.org/health/wellness-and-prevention/acupuncture

*Mayo Clinic Article on Acupuncture*
https://www.mayoclinic.org/tests-procedures/acupuncture/about/pac-20392763

*Memorial Sloan Kettering Description of Acupuncture*
https://www.mskcc.org/cancer-care/integrative-medicine/therapies/acupuncture

*Medical News Today Article on Acupuncture*
https://www.medicalnewstoday.com/articles/156488

*National Library of Medicine section on Traditional Chinese Medicine*
https://www.nlm.nih.gov/hmd/topics/chinese-traditional/index.html

*National Multiple Sclerosis Society Explanation of Acupuncture*
https://www.nationalmssociety.org/Treating-MS/Complementary-Alternative-Medicines/Acupuncture

*NIH/NCCIH Description of Acupuncture*
https://www.nccih.nih.gov/health/
acupuncture-what-you-need-to-know

*Sacred Lotus Chinese Medicine*
https://www.sacredlotus.com/

*VA Whole Health System Use of Acupuncture*
https://www.va.gov/WHOLEHEALTH/professional-resources/
Acupuncture.asp

*WebMD Slideshow: A Visual Guide to Acupuncture*
https://www.webmd.com/pain-management/ss/
slideshow-acupuncture-overview

## Acupuncture-Related Organizations in the United States

*Accreditation Commission for Acupuncture and Herbal Medicine (ACAHM)*
https://acahm.org/

*Acupuncture Now Foundation*
https://acupuncturenowfoundation.org

*American Academy of Medical Acupuncture*
https://medicalacupuncture.org/

*American Association of Acupuncture and Oriental Medicine (AAAOM)*

https://www.aaaomonline.org/

*American Association of Chinese Medicine and Acupuncture (AACMA)*

https://www.aacmaonline.com/en/

*American Association of Traditional Chinese Medicine Alumni Associations (TCMAAA)*

https://www-tcmaaa-org.translate.goog/en/home/?_x_tr_sl=zh-CN&_x_tr_tl=en&_x_tr_hl=en&_x_tr_pto=sc&_x_tr_sch=http

*American Society of Acupuncturists (ASA)*

https://www.asacu.org/

*American Traditional Chinese Medicine Association (ATCMA)*

https://atcma-us.org/

*Council for Higher Education Accreditation link to ACAHM*

https://www.chea.org/
accreditation-commission-acupuncture-and-herbal-medicine

*Council of Colleges of Acupuncture and Herbal Medicine (CCAHM)*

https://www.ccahm.org/ccaom/default.asp

*National Certification Commission for Acupuncture and Oriental Medicine (NCCAOM)*

https://pedr.nccaom.org/#!

*National Federations of Chinese TCM Organizations (NFCTCMO)*
https://www.nfctcmo.org/

*Society for Acupuncture Research (SAR)*
https://www.acupunctureresearch.org/

*World Federation of Chinese Medicine Societies (WFCMS)*
https://www.wcprtcm.org/

# ACKNOWLEDGMENTS

I am grateful to the following people for helping to make this book possible. I would like to thank my writing partner, Marla, for sitting next to me in the coffee shop week after week and forcing me—gently and by her excellent example—to keep my nose in my computer and my fingers on the keyboard. Accountability is everything. Larry, I am so grateful to you for jumping in and creating a beautiful cradle to house my words. You are a true master of your craft, and everything you touch is beautiful. To my coach, Kemia, thank you for your unwavering support and consistent wisdom.

I am grateful to the following people for helping make this book better. Thank you to Johanna and Charlotte, who offered constructive feedback on the very first draft and encouragement right from the start. Thank you to Kim for helping me soften my emphatic nature and to Martha for helping me see that this could actually be a good enough book to keep you from doing your chores. A particularly large thank you goes to Saskia, who is not only a remarkably fast reader but also an astute listener of what I was trying to say. As always, you helped me to say it better. Thank you to Lil, who spoke up and gave me a chance with GWN Publishing when I was feeling in over my head.

Thank you, Mark, for the time, encouragement, and space to dream that this would be possible and for supporting me at every step along the way. And for letting me interrupt whatever you were doing to ask you to listen to me read that paragraph aloud again or to brainstorm with me about how to tackle a tricky phrase. And for sensing when I needed a break and when I needed to keep going. And for assuming I had forgotten to eat and just bringing me soup. And for being proud of me. I love being married to you, and I'm so grateful every day for your presence in my life.

Thank you to all the people who have listened to me say the book will be done next week and who just nodded and smiled instead of reminding me that I said that last week. It is an ongoing lesson of mine to be patient with myself...and to not set myself on fire to keep other people (or myself) warm. Thank you for being my gracious, compassionate teachers.

Finally, thank you to all the people who were brave enough and curious enough to ask these questions of me. In so doing, you have allowed me to practice answering your questions over many years. By the time I got to the place where I started writing this book, you had already helped me to craft what I might say and how I might say it. I am so deeply grateful. Thank you.

# ABOUT THE AUTHOR

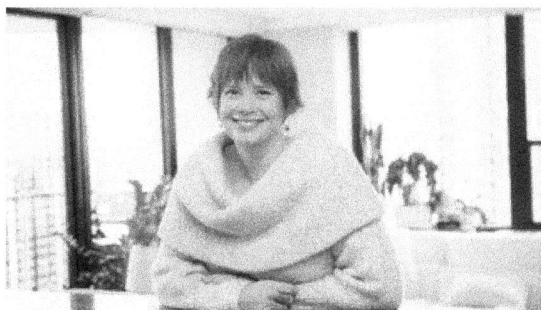

*Dr. Sina Smith* is a medical doctor who was at the end of her general surgery training when pain and paralysis of her arm led her to find acupuncture. She attended school to become a licensed acupuncturist and trained extensively in a variety of other integrative healing modalities, after which she worked in multiple academic and private settings. Dr. Smith has dedicated herself to educating patients and fellow clinicians in natural healing methods. Out of that dedication, she has written "Demystifying Acupuncture," her first book.

www.ingramcontent.com/pod-product-compliance
Lightning Source LLC
Chambersburg PA
CBHW070110030426
42335CB00016B/2086